No Ordinary Love Story

No Ordinary Love Story

SOPHIE MORGAN

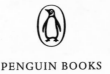

PENGUIN BOOKS

PENGUIN BOOKS

Published by the Penguin Group
Penguin Books Ltd, 80 Strand, London WC2R ORL, England
Penguin Group (USA) Inc., 375 Hudson Street, New York, New York 10014, USA
Penguin Group (Canada), 90 Eglinton Avenue East, Suite 700, Toronto, Ontario, Canada M4P 2Y3
(a division of Pearson Penguin Canada Inc.)
Penguin Ireland, 25 St Stephen's Green, Dublin 2, Ireland (a division of Penguin Books Ltd)
Penguin Group (Australia), 707 Collins Street, Melbourne, Victoria 3008, Australia
(a division of Pearson Australia Group Pty Ltd)
Penguin Books India Pvt Ltd, 11 Community Centre, Panchsheel Park, New Delhi – 110 017, India
Penguin Group (NZ), 67 Apollo Drive, Rosedale, Auckland 0632, New Zealand
(a division of Pearson New Zealand Ltd)
Penguin Books (South Africa) (Pty) Ltd, Block D, Rosebank Office Park,
181 Jan Smuts Avenue, Parktown North, Gauteng 2193, South Africa

Penguin Books Ltd, Registered Offices: 80 Strand, London WC2R ORL, England

www.penguin.com

First published in Great Britain in Penguin Books 2013
001

Copyright © Sophie Morgan 2013

Printed in England by Clays Ltd, St Ives plc

ISBN: 978-1-405-91282-2

www.greenpenguin.co.uk

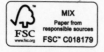

ALWAYS LEARNING   **PEARSON**

For F, with all my love and thanks

Chapter One

I was late. I spend a lot of my life late, or if not actually late then in fear of being so. I'm a journalist, and work-wise while it's an occupational hazard there's nothing less forgivable (OK, except maybe phone hacking, but I'm a local newspaper journalist so that's not the kind of thing we get up to, whatever you might see in the soaps). In my non-work life I find lateness annoying in myself and in others. Wherever possible I'll pitch up five minutes early and loiter just to minimise the risk of being late. I know I probably look a bit like a stalker, but that's a price I'm willing to pay.

No chance to do that this time, though. When I got to the bar my friends, Thomas and Charlotte, had already commandeered a booth and were waving at me like luna-tics to get me to come over. Charlotte was even wearing an elf hat, which is not as odd as it sounds as it was four days before Christmas. The festive spirit had completely passed me by, though, partly because work was bedlam and partly because I was still licking my wounds over the longest break-up ever. The only reason I'd agreed to come for drinks was because I couldn't cope with their lecturing if I declined. Plus, the bar was close to my office and Charlotte had assured me there would be lots of people – enough I hoped for me to be able to slip away unnoticed after a quick drink and some mingling to show willing and shut them up. Except as I walked over to the bar I realised that there was only one other person in the booth with them. I'd been ambushed.

My first thought, testament to how he was still not really ever out of my mind, was that it was James, my ex, even though rationally I knew Thomas wasn't ever going to be sharing drinks, small talk and mini cheesy biscuits with him. I wasn't actually sure I wanted to share drinks with him either. The man with his back to me turned round, confirming what I knew, and then the annoyance began to burn in the pit of my stomach. I couldn't have told you who I was angry at – myself? Them? Him? I'd spent a lot of time angry lately. It was unlike me and I was beginning to bore myself with it. It was also exhausting, another reason I would have been happier sitting at home watching cooking shows on TV and not speaking to anyone.

No chance of that tonight, though. I'd been completely stitched up by my so-called friends. Charlotte hesitated for a moment before she hugged me, able to see my rage, but Thomas showed no such fear. He launched himself at me and enveloped me in a massive bear hug that almost made me overbalance.

'Soph! You made it. We didn't think you were going to come, it's not like you to be late.'

I slipped out of his arms and began unbuttoning my coat. 'Yeah, work was a pain and the tube was packed.' I had no intention of apologising for my lateness. I bit back a wry smile, remembering an occasion when, upon turning up at Thomas's twenty-three minutes late due to traffic trouble, he hit me twenty-three times with a crop. It felt like a long time ago, a different life. Things really had changed, although the memory still inspired a surge of affection which went some way to easing my fury.

The-man-who-wasn't-James had stood up as I arrived and was waiting for me to come closer to the table. As I leaned in to put my coat on the pile he put his hand out.

'Hello, Sophie. I'm Adam. It's lovely to meet you, I've heard so much about you.' Dark hair, brown eyes, glasses. Strong handshake, nice hands – I notice these things; it's a side effect of my extra-curricular love of spanking. I had to give them credit for knowing my tastes well. Shame they didn't know me well enough to know I had no interest in any kind of relationship with anyone for the foreseeable future.

'Have you really?' I smiled at him, not entirely sure it was reaching my eyes. 'Because I've heard nothing at all about you.' I glanced over at Charlotte, who looked discomfited. The silence lengthened, and for a moment I let it hang there, before sighing, plonking myself down on the cushioned bench and picking up the menu. I hate confrontations and bad atmospheres, I always have. I could play nice; all I had to do was get through the next hour or so and cry off with an early work start. My eyes caught mulled wine on the menu and I smiled to myself. I could get a little bit into the festive spirit at least. 'So what's everyone drinking? I'll get them.'

I know I sound a bit churlish, and I know it wasn't poor Adam's fault. The fact is, and I appreciate this sounds all

3

Mills & Boon, I'd had my heart broken not long before. Not on purpose – people who break your heart on purpose are the worst kind of bastards after all, and if I'd found myself in love with a bastard it'd have been much easier to disentangle my life, pull myself together and move on. But James had managed to pretty much settle his way into my life, both as a boyfriend and as a dominant foil to my submissive tendencies. Then he ended things abruptly and it had left me feeling uncharacteristically adrift.

Not that things had ended completely, not in a way I had been able to start moving on from yet. If I was to describe this in a TV-style 'previously on Sophie's life' segment then the admittedly HBO-friendly summary is as follows: Boy meets girl, boy dominates girl, girl gets off on the pain and degradation and falls for boy, boy becomes guilt-ridden at how he's dominating the girl he's decided he's in love with, girl points out she enjoys the domination. You'd imagine the next step would be boy coming to terms with the two sides of his nature and thanking his lucky stars he had found a girl that complemented him so well but, alas, that hadn't happened. After weeks of text messages – flurries of affection and emotional chat which made the silence immediately afterwards ever more distressing – I'd decided it was time to stop, for my own sanity. I asked one last time if anything could work between us and, taking his silence as a pretty strong answer, I changed my phone number and set a filter on my email account that automatically forwarded any messages he sent me to the trash. Hell, after the first week or two I stopped checking three times a day in case there *had*

4

been any automatically deleted messages. That was progress, right?

I was trying, slowly, to move on. But it hurt. And I felt stupid. So stupid. So for now I was happy to be on my own. If nothing else it meant as few people as possible got wind of my idiocy.

I knew now more than ever that my love of sexual submission was something that I definitely wanted as part of any relationship – only part, admittedly, but for me a lack of that basic compatibility was a deal-breaker. But having realised that, and then being let down by James so badly when he turned out to be a bit emotionally stunted, I'd decided that it was time to take a step back for a bit. Because while sexual compatibility was an important aspect of the kind of relationship I wanted, it was part of a bigger whole – I wanted someone caring, clever, funny, who put up with my obsession with TV (and the associated stacks of DVD box sets), loved their job enough that they didn't get annoyed at how hard I worked at mine, and had similar ideas on life in the long term, i.e. one day getting married and having kids.

I know. I want the moon on a bloody stick. And the thing is, finding a bloke who ticked a lot of those boxes (not ALL of them, I'm not that unreasonable), was a dominant and who wanted a woman like me, well that's the equivalent of winning the relationship lottery. And right now, after my disappointment with James, I didn't even want to buy a ticket and then suffer the disappointment. Not least because I was hardly ankle deep in dominant sorts – if there was such a thing as kinky radar then I most definitely didn't have it, and even with my sexual proclivities I drew the line at randomly asking guys if they'd like to hurt me. Let's face it, the sort of guys that would say yes were probably the kind you should be crossing the street to avoid anyway. I'd used online D/s sites before, to chat to folk and make friends, but I wasn't ready to start the time-consuming and occasionally soul-destroying search for a date on them yet – even though one of my best friends, and ex-dom, Thomas had found his current squeeze by doing just that.

Nope, I was getting my kicks through an erotica-packed Kindle and not much else lately and I was fine with that. I just didn't feel I had the energy for anything more, especially through the always-manic festive season. I had it all planned. I'd been taking on as much overtime as work would give me, sitting through more out-of-hours council meetings than any sane person should ever want to. I'd booked time off to head home to my parents for the Christmas holidays. I was working New Year's Eve and New Year's Day. I was filling my life with work and reading and sleep, and that was fine.

Unfortunately bloody Charlotte and Tom didn't seem to think it *was* fine.

I drank my mulled wine as fast as I was able to without burning the roof of my mouth, and excused myself to go to the loo, rehearsing the explanation I'd give for having to leave early on my way back. But when I got back to the table Charlotte had bought me another glass in my absence. My 'thank you' for it was through gritted teeth and she couldn't meet my eyes when I looked at her, but even in my most antisocial of modes I wouldn't have buggered off and left then. I drank it – a bit slower this time – and resigned myself to listening to the conversation washing over me.

Adam was interesting. Funny. Clever. Witty. Self-deprecating. He had quite a way with words and enjoyed using puns, presumably in part due to his career as a copywriter. He was exactly the kind of person I would have enjoyed spending time with normally. Not so tonight, though. I know this makes me stubborn, but, while I liked him, I had no intention of showing that to him or – more importantly – Charlotte and Thomas, who clearly thought they knew better than me what I needed, and seemed to be suffering from a small case of that irritating condition where couples insist on trying to pair off all their single friends. Even if Adam was happy to stand for that, I really wasn't.

He was good company, though. As a group we chatted about TV that we'd all been watching, recommending shows to each other, with him suggesting I pick up the DVDs of *The Shield*, a police show that had completely passed me by but which was made by one of the guys behind another show I had loved, *Lie to Me*. He told a great anecdote about a political campaign he'd worked on, which meant before I knew it I was sharing similar war stories from events I'd covered. I found myself leaning in to talk to him, catching myself and then deliberately moving back to feign indifference.

I finally finished my drink and headed home. My fury had eased a little, but I was still slightly stand-offish with Charlotte and Thomas as I said goodbye. I waved at Adam as I left, not even wanting to encourage their meddling by kissing him on the cheek in farewell lest it was misconstrued.

By the time I got home and was curled up in my current non-work default position – on the sofa in my PJs with a mug of tea and the late news – my phone had pinged several times.

Charlotte and Thomas had both texted, ostensibly to check I'd got home OK, but both with variants of 'Sorry if you felt slightly ambushed'. I wasn't forgiving them easily. I also had a Facebook notification: Adam had tracked me down and sent me a message.

I harrumphed slightly to myself as I opened it on my phone. This was exactly the kind of faff I could do without.

From: Adam
To: Sophie

I wanted to send you a brief note to apologise for tonight. Not for meeting you (that was fun) but for the fact that clearly you weren't expecting me to be there when you arrived.

I broke up with my long-term girlfriend fairly recently and I think Charlotte was trying to encourage me to find someone new in her usual sledgehammer-like fashion. Please rest assured I'm not the sort of person to get dates under false pretences – apologies for any awkwardness.

Best,
Adam

Suddenly it all made sense. I could kick Charlotte. In her head this must have felt brilliant – two of her single friends hooking up – but now I felt even more awkward. 'Best'? Ouch. I smiled wryly to myself for being such an egotist – so much for *me* being such a big catch!

From: Sophie
To: Adam

Bloody Charlotte! I'm so sorry. I didn't stop to think that it might be as awkward for you too – I fear you handled it better. I might have come across a smidgen grumpy. Sorry. It definitely wasn't personal.

I hope Charlotte's attempts at 'helping' haven't made your break-up feel any more rotten than they tend to.

Sophie
PS Fear not, you don't look like the sort to need to get dates under duress.

His reply was quick, intriguing and made it obvious that he wasn't any more interested in me than I was in him.

From: Adam
To: Sophie

Break-up was a long time coming and as painless as these things can be. We dated for a year pretty much to the day and had a lot of fun but fundamentally wanted different things – she loves travelling and wanted to work her way around America. I like holidays, but wanted to stay closer to home long term for marriage, kids etc. One of those things. She sent me a mail tonight actually. She's currently working as a receptionist in a tattoo parlour in San Francisco somewhere. We're both OK. It's just the thing with break-ups – everyone assumes you want to be straight back in a relationship again. Sometimes it's nice to have a break.

A

PS You were a little grumpy. It was oddly endearing though.
I didn't take it personally.

I chuckled to myself.

From: Sophie
To: Adam

I hear you on the 'break from relationships' front. Sometimes life
is simpler being single.

Soph.

I shut down my laptop, fairly sure that would be the last I heard of him and happy that I'd made it clear I wasn't interested in any overtures, even if any were forthcoming. Little did I know.

The next morning he sent me a message linking me to a news story about the politician we'd been discussing the night before. Before I knew it I'd tapped a brief message back. He replied, asking at the same time if I'd heard from a more-apologetic Charlotte (I had). I replied asking if he'd had anything to do with her new-found regret (he did). Suddenly we were emailing at least a couple of times a day.

It was safe. It was simple. We talked about non-contentious things: my mum's internet-fuelled holiday planning (military invasions have taken less work), his trip to Yorkshire for a family wedding. I tracked down and watched (although admittedly from behind my hands at points) a couple of episodes of *The Shield* at his behest and was blown away by it, but had no one else to wax lyrical about it with, so we enthused about that. I recommended a couple of political biographies which had passed him by. All in all it was surprisingly fun to chat.

I also (don't judge me) took advantage of the fact that his Facebook privacy settings were much less locked down than mine and checked out his profile. I looked at some of his pictures (mostly holidays, family trips and parties) and skim read his most recent updates – mostly links to news stories with associated rants, comments about TV shows and films he'd just seen and geeky internet memes, all of which I found very interesting, although I didn't dare so much as 'like' anything lest Charlotte or Thomas see and get the wrong idea. That first step of modern interaction – friending him on Facebook – was also a definite no-no.

Then one night the tone of things changed a little. By this point we were chatting on Messenger some evenings if we were both around – OK, if he was in, because I was still under voluntary non-work house arrest. We'd been discussing another attempt by some of his friends to set him up – this time with a secondary school physics teacher. I'd been laughing quietly to myself at his obvious horror at the awkward small talk, when suddenly a line of what he'd written caught my eye.

> Adam says: The thing is there's no good way to have that discussion about compatibility is there? At least Charlotte put US together knowing we had complementary personalities on that front!

I sat up straighter, my heart beginning to pound a bit. My fingers were a flurry, and then stopped. Did he mean what I thought he meant or was I being over-sensitive? Obviously Charlotte knew I was submissive, by first-hand experience in fact. But would she really have told some guy I'd never met? I was torn between asking for clarification and accidentally outing myself when in fact she hadn't done any such thing. In the end curiosity won out.

Sophie says: Complementary personalities how?

His reply confirmed my fears.

*Adam says: Sexually I mean. It's not a prerequisite for a
relationship, but it's definitely something when it feels right to
start dating again that I'd like to factor into things.*

I have a tendency to set off on occasional flights of fancy. I can't help it. Eventually my rational brain does kick in but for now my thoughts were whirring. He knew I was a sub. Had known from the beginning. Was this some kind of ridiculous long-game thing? Did he think I was playing hard to get? How could Charlotte have told him that without telling me? I was incandescent with rage.

The sudden silence at my end seemingly spoke volumes.

Adam says: Sophie?

I cast my laptop aside to grab a drink from the kitchen, not sure what, if anything, I should say in reply. When I got back the screen was filled with text.

*Adam says: I've not made you uncomfortable mentioning it
have I? I promise it's not a thing. Charlie just mentioned in
passing that we both met her at the same place independent
of each other. She didn't tell me anything else about you, but
I figured that she'd only set us up if you were submissive or at
least switch. Apologies if I've stepped out of line.*

Thomas and I had met Charlotte at a munch – a kind
of social get-together for kinky folk (rest assured, there
was no leather and chains, it was just a meeting in a pub).
If he'd met her in the same place . . . Oh.

Suddenly my brain was whirring with questions – I was
curious, having never thought of Adam in those kind of
terms. I guess you really should be careful about making
assumptions about people. I knew he must be dominant,
given he'd assumed I was submissive or switch (someone
who both dominates and submits).

*Sophie says: It's OK, I'm not uncomfortable. Surprised you
knew. I didn't know that about you. It just put me on the
back foot a bit. It's fine.*

I wondered if I'd over-egged it. Even to my ears it
didn't sound 'fine'. Sod it. Bloody Charlotte. Also, damn
my curiosity because now more than anything I wanted to
know about him.

Sophie says: So do you go to munches a lot?

I know. I'm incredibly nosey. But I was also curious –
not least because I'd not pegged him as especially dominant.

13

Definitely no kinky radar (should we call it kaydar?) here, although admittedly when I met him I wasn't looking at him in any sexual terms at all, soulful eyes or not.

Adam says: I did for a while. It's where I met Kathryn, my ex. She was a sub. Haven't been to one for a while though. Despite what you might now worry, to the contrary I'm really not angling to start dating again. Sorry I brought this up though if it feels awkward.

I had a moment of realisation. Now I knew that Charlotte hadn't been telling him the intimate details of what we'd got up to together it actually felt OK.

Sophie says: It's not awkward. It's fine. I was just surprised, that's all. Charlotte didn't mention it.

His reply was quick.

Adam says: She's terrible that one. She means well though.

I knew he was right, but I still felt inclined to give her a stern talking to at a later date. Before I could reply, another message pinged through.

Adam says: One last question before we move back to non D/s stuff if that's OK?

Sophie says: I'm not sure I should answer this, but go on . . .

Somewhat inevitably, it wasn't the last time we talked about D/s. Slowly, over a period of weeks and for the first time in ages, I chatted to someone about kink without there being any underlying subtext to it. Neither of us had any expectations. We were both adamant we didn't want to date. There was no hint that this would become anything, or that we'd get together. It was just nice to chat about life with someone for whom the kink side of things wasn't unusual – it could be mentioned in passing without it being a big or defining thing.

He told me how he'd had lots of kinky fun with his girl-friend, but their relationship had floundered because they didn't have much in common bar their interest in sex. I told him a little about what had happened with James and his insight and kindness was a balm to my emotional bruises.

In flirtier chats – admittedly often late at night – we discussed some of our experiences. Not in explicit terms, but more generally and in enough depth that I was intrigued as to what kind of a dominant he would be. It was apparent he'd had a lot more D/s experience than me and that his interest was as much about the mental aspect of domination as physically inflicting pain. I found it intriguing. I found him intriguing. But he was also incredibly gentlemanly. He was respectful and thoughtful when we spoke – whether about general day-to-day stuff or in-depth emotional things.

Every so often one or other of us would make a passing comment about how we should meet for a drink, but we never got round to sorting it out, initially using the busy New Year period as an excuse, although by that time we were well into January. I took his lack of initiative as a sign he wasn't interested in me that way, which of course should have been a relief. At points, though, it didn't feel that way. I wasn't sure I should feel insulted, but, in typically contrary terms, I most definitely did.

Why wasn't he interested in me romantically? What was I, chopped liver?

I know, I'm a lunatic. But it was just a thought. I kept it to myself. Then one day we were discussing Charlotte's latest attempts to get him to go to a munch with her and Tom. What *was* it with her trying to hook him up anyway?

Adam says: I told her I wasn't interested and she tried to convince me that it was worth going just to find someone to let off some steam with.

Sophie says: 'Let off some steam with'? Sounds a bit clinical.

Adam says: I know. Don't get me wrong, sometimes I like the idea of some no-strings fun, but I want it to be with someone I have at least some connection with and know is going to be laid-back about it. I don't want to end up with someone feeling like I'm just using them for sex.

Sophie says: You want to have fun with someone who isn't up for a relationship either and thus you're not leading on?

Adam says: Exactly.

Sophie says: Someone whose feelings you aren't inadvertently going to hurt because they end up wanting more?

Adam says: Yes.

Sophie says: Someone into the same things you're into, who is up for experimenting and having some fun but will still be doing their own thing?

Adam says: Yes, that's it.

I bet you can see where this is going. I didn't; I wasn't even conscious of my fingers moving until I'd tapped out the message and hit send.

Sophie says: Someone like me?

Fuck. As soon as I said it I wished I could take it back. What was I thinking? I know I hadn't had any kind of sex with anyone in months, much less had any D/s-ish fun, but he wasn't interested in me that way. Shit. Now this was awkward. I began trying to type something, *anything*, that would make it sound like what I'd written was a joke, but before I could finish the sentence his reply flashed up.

Adam says: Yes, someone exactly like you.

Oh.

Chapter Two

The thing is, saying something in the heat of the moment and then having the courage or inclination to actually do it are two slightly different things. I'll admit it, reading Adam's reply made me smile to myself and feel a little bit giddy, not least because it proved the growing text-based attraction between us wasn't (all) one way. But it didn't mean we shut down our laptops and he came flying round so we could fuck fifteen ways to Sunday. It's not that I have any moral issue with that – hell, we'd chatted enough that we knew each other better than the average couple hooking up in a club on a Saturday night. But I was cautious. And, I was realising, so was he. And maybe it's a bit crazy, but that knowledge actually made me feel reassured, especially after falling so far so fast for James.

I honestly didn't know how to reply to his message. Feeling lost for words was very uncharacteristic for me, but in the days that followed it became a recurring theme of my chats with Adam.

Adam says: I'm sorry if you think this is maybe a bit forward (ha, how BBC period drama of me) but I really do like you, I think you're sparky and interesting and as we've chatted I've come to the realisation I would like to do rude things with you. And to you.

Sophie says: That probably is a bit forward, but I'll let you off. Although best you didn't say that to me in person. At least this way you can't see me blush.

Adam says: I want to see you blush.

I was torn. My head still said I wasn't ready to try any kind of relationship again, much less in the market for a 'with benefits' arrangement. But my heart (and, OK, places a fair bit lower) found Adam fun and sexy and, as his messages got flirtier as the days passed, I increasingly thought, 'Well why not'?

He didn't push for an answer about us meeting, but we ended up having increasingly rude chats. In hindsight it felt like it was a mixture of him giving me an insight into the fun we could have together and intriguing me enough to want to try. What helped was, as a copywriter, he was incredibly creative when he chatted about things we could do (somewhere along the way our chats had moved from things we had done or might like to do to things we might like to do together) and I increasingly found myself lying in bed at night thinking of the scenarios he had woven. They were definitely hot thoughts.

The conversation still ebbed and flowed between kink and real life. One week I had two busy days complete with evening jobs and our email exchanges were brief and purely about news stories developing through the day. But then on the third day I opened an email from him and found lengthy paragraphs – he'd turned a casual comment I'd made about fantasising about having sex outside into a full-length story with us as the protagonists.

It took a couple of seconds for me to realise that, though. I was sitting at my desk at work, and as I scanned down the message I found myself beginning to flush bright red. I closed the email in case anyone in our open-plan office could read it over my shoulder.

He then sent me a separate message, asking me if I'd liked the story. I told him that I hadn't read it properly yet, but had been given a bit of a shock getting it out of the blue while in the office. His response suggested I should potentially be worried about his interest in embarrass-ing me.

Adam says: Did it make you blush?

I felt my lips twitch into a smile even while I still felt the warmth on my cheeks. As if I was going to tell him that.

Sophie says: Knob.

OK, maybe in hindsight I actually had just told him that . . .

After what felt like the longest afternoon in the world I finally got home from work and read his story. It was incredible. The scenario was hot and it was really well written (I know that shouldn't be a major factor, but trust me, for me it was). By the time I got to the end my hand had slipped inside my knickers.

Interestingly, he'd focused a lot on the female sub's point of view, exploring her thoughts. Mostly that was the kind of erotica I enjoyed anyway, but over and above that

I found his choice of style interesting – his insights into the shifts of fear and excitement, and his understanding and explanation of her mindset showed he was clearly very perceptive, and that made me more intrigued at the kind of dominant he might be, how he would control me. It also, of course, made me think about how easily he might be able to understand and respond to my own reactions if we did anything together. He was definitely clever.

After I'd finished reading I logged in to Messenger and sent him a message.

> *Sophie says: I've finally had some privacy to read it, and just wanted to say thanks so much for the story. It was amazing. No one's ever written anything like that for me before (possibly the occupational hazard of being a writer by trade).*
>
> *Adam says: You're very welcome. I'm glad you enjoyed it. Did it make you wet?*

My fingers stilled over the keys. Of course it had made me wet. We both knew that. Why was typing out that it had so difficult? This really didn't bode well for challenges in person.

> *Sophie says: Yes it did.*
>
> *Adam says: Good.*

From that point our chats on Messenger shifted a little further along the axis of smut. He didn't make demands or act like some kind of überdom, but he made oh-so-polite requests that I found increasingly difficult to turn down – and while I mentally cursed the need to please so inherent in my personality, I knew it was more than that. Increasingly, I wanted to please *him*.

I wrote him a story too, channelling a lot of the thoughts I had lying in bed at night about the kind of things we could get up to together. He sent me a message saying how much he enjoyed it and how hard it had made him, both of which made me feel butterflies. Then he suggested some things we could also do in the scenario I'd sketched out and suddenly we were having creative, filthy chat.

It was huge amounts of fun. Nothing was off limits, and – in part because of Adam's easy-going openness and in part because our friendship was relatively new and thus it didn't feel like a huge risk to say something rude that might disturb him forever – we could talk about anything: fantasies, limits and the like. It was a new level of communication for me and it was really lovely and liberating. It was often illuminating too, for example when it became apparent that we were both quite laid-back in our attitudes about D/s.

> *Adam says: I find this whole rigmarole of being called Master or Sir a bit embarrassing really. You shouldn't need to call me a special name to show me respect in that context.*

Before I'd even begun typing a reply, a second comment pinged in.

> *Adam says: I love D/s and the whole dynamic, but I'm not the sort of guy that wants to live it all the time. I know some people love the idea of a completely obedient and subservient*

submissive, but to be honest I find that a bit boring. For me submissive can't mean passive. There needs to be some spark. Partly it's about the challenge – how do I get you to do what I want you to? What will you respond to? But partly it's also because I want to enjoy being with someone – arguing about politics or doing something (other than sex) we're both passionate about. The challenge is where it gets fun, in whatever context that is.

His messages made me smile. They also eased my mind a bit – his motivations chimed very much with my own, and his ideas on the kind of sub he liked fitted well with me. I liked him but I knew I wasn't going to be the 'eyes permanently downcast, referring to herself in the third person' kind of submissive that some dominants liked. He wasn't interested in that either. Phew. I was already pretty sure he didn't have a problem with being disagreed with and mocked, but it's always good to know for sure.

Sophie says: Ironically enough, I enjoy the challenge of submission. I can't decide if this means we're really compatible or at odds.

Adam says: Can't it be both? It could definitely be an interesting experience.

We discussed my limits (and his – another comfort; I'd never been with a dominant who'd talked much about his own limits, the implications being that it didn't matter). He asked how I would feel about breath play and face slapping – I had limited experience of the latter and was intrigued by the former, but explained that while I was curious about both and found them hot in the abstract they were things I was concerned about trying for the first time.

Adam says: Don't worry. We won't leap into lots of new things. If we do this we'll take things slow and steady.

I felt reassured.

We chatted like this every night for a few weeks, driving each other a bit loopy with lust, although it wasn't all sex talk – sometimes we just exchanged thoughts while watching the same TV show in our respective flats. Then one day he said he had a big night out the next evening with his friends and wouldn't be around to chat.

I admit it, the thought of not speaking to him felt weird, but I told him to have a good time and that I'd speak to him the following day. Not talking to him made me feel strangely out of sorts, though, and my resolution to leave him in peace and not text and email (no, not even the link to that hilarious cartoon that I'd just read but which could keep until the morning) was tough to stick to.

But at about 7.30 p.m. my phone pinged and I realised it wasn't just me finding it difficult. It was a text from Adam:

> Hey gorgeous. How're you
> doing? Did you get back
> from your meeting ok? X

I practically hugged myself with the knowledge that he was thinking of me. Lame? Yes. But I did.

> I'm good. Got back a while
> ago, now just watching TV and
> having dinner. X

I know it wasn't the most riveting of texts, but it was true, plus I wasn't trying to pull him into a long conversation while he was out with his friends, remember?

In the next hour he texted a few times. As time passed, his messages became more frequent.

> I know you might think it's the
> beer talking, but I'm missing
> talking to you tonight. Filth
> and otherwise. X

I replied (secretly thinking it probably was the beer talking, but if there was one thing my university years taught me it was never argue with a drunk person when you're sober), saying that I felt the same way but that he should concentrate on socialising with his friends. He replied quickly, pointing out it was a big group and there was lots of chat going on so it wasn't especially rude. I wasn't convinced (but I'm the sort of person that bristles if someone gets their phone out while at a restaurant unless they're an on-call doctor, leader of the free world or some such) but at the same time I was chuffed that he still wanted to chat. And he really did. His spelling got a bit worse the more he drank and his language got dirtier, but by the end he was most definitely, in newspaper parlance, sexting.

It was hot, made oddly hotter by the fact he was sat in a group in the pub unable to do anything while I was comfortably curled up on the sofa in a convenient place to deal with any lustful urges. He'd just sent me a message detailing pinching my nipples when I had a surge of inspiration on how to take advantage of that difference in social setting. I used my camera phone to take a picture of my breasts, showing how hard my nipples were.

Now, I'm not (too) foolish. I deleted the picture afterwards and my face wasn't in it – not, I hasten to add, because I had any particular concerns about trusting Adam, but more because if either one of us lost our phones I didn't want pictures of me grinning with my baps out available to any random person who found the handset.

When my phone pinged, telling me I had another message, I felt a bit nervous before I read it. I'd just sent him a picture of my breasts on their own for goodness' sake. Who finds that hot? What if his friends had seen? The message opened.

You're incredible. X

I couldn't decide if he was talking specifically about my breasts or my new-found propensity for sexting, but either way as compliments went I was happy with that.

As you might expect, things got hotter and ruder from that point on as the night progressed. Finally I got a text saying he was home, feeling a bit drunk but lying in bed, relieved that – finally – he was able to touch himself at last.

After a smart-arse message about how I was impressed with his self-restraint, but it was probably a good thing as otherwise he might have disturbed his cab driver, suddenly my phone trilled into life.

This wasn't a text message. He was ringing me.

I know, it's bonkers for me to have felt awkward about that, but I really did. I answered with some trepidation. Maybe it's daft, maybe it's a sign of my confidence in the written word, but actually talking to him felt a bit embarrassing after all the rude texts. Typing was definitely easier.

The first thing I thought when he said hello was that I'd forgotten (or maybe not noticed at all) how lovely his voice was. Deep, soothing. The second thing I thought, with not a little relief, was that while he sounded tired he didn't sound completely shit-faced. Always a relief. Actually, he was very coherent and rather creative with the dirty things he started saying to me. At his suggestion, I slipped my hand into my knickers as we talked and I soon felt my orgasm approaching. He must have heard my breathing change, because suddenly his voice was in my ear with the worst kind of inopportune statement.

'Don't come yet please, Sophie.'

What? Was he kidding? I asked him to repeat what he'd just said. Alas, I hadn't misheard.

I held off as long as I could, changing the movements of my fingers, but frankly it was a difficult one, not least because we'd been driving each other crazy for hours by this point.

Finally he spoke again, asking me to come now, to come with him. I wasn't even sure what he meant as my orgasm washed over me, but then I heard his groan and realised. It made me smile.

We chatted into the early hours after that. Some kink

stuff, some life stuff. It was nice, made me feel this wasn't all about us getting our rocks off. Although a great part of it was, and that was OK too.

Finally he asked me if I would consider some no-strings D/s fun with him. My concerns had been eased through our chats and I knew what my answer would be. That didn't mean it wasn't fun to play with him a little before I answered.

'That's hardly a fair question to ask someone after they've just had an orgasm.'

He laughed, and it felt warm and intimate and made me smile in the darkness of my bedroom. 'It's better to ask afterwards than before I let you come.'

I tutted. 'Actually, you didn't "let me", it wasn't about permission. You asked me to wait and I did. You're not my dom just yet.'

'Yet.' I couldn't work out if he was agreeing with me or pointing out the implicit agreement in my words. 'You're right, I asked you. Of course I might not be so polite if I actually were your dom.'

My heart began beating faster just at the thought of it. Right, let's do this.

'Maybe we should find out.'

We began making plans for him to come round the following weekend.

So what *is* the etiquette when someone's coming round your house just for sex? Should I get wine in? Would he want dinner? Would he consider food an unwelcome distraction? My brain was a frenzy of indecision through the whole day. It was a Sunday. He'd gone for lunch with his family to celebrate a birthday and we'd arranged for him to head over in the early evening. I, notionally, had the day off work but after a few hours buzzing round my flat getting increasingly nervous I decided to nip into the office for a bit to write up a couple of interviews before heading to the shop to buy whatever I had decided was socially appropriate food and beverages.

In the end I bought wine and decided to bake chocolate chip cookies in case he wanted tea. I'd hoped that the precision of the baking, the creaming and stirring, which I'd done dozens of times before would calm me down, soothe me and let me switch my brain off. What I should have done was gone for something exotic that I'd never made before and that I had to concentrate on, because what I found instead was my mind was wandering, trying to piece together the things I knew about him, the things he'd hinted at being into, to try and get a feel for the kind of man – the kind of dominant – he would be, which of course threw up comparisons with dominants I'd been with previously.

For the first time in a while I'd gone through all the pre-date rituals that make me feel comfortable before someone sees me naked – the shaving and plucking and buffing and moisturising. It made me feel pangs, knowing the last time I'd prepared myself so extensively for fucking had been for James on that last and most intense weekend, the memories of which still replayed in my dreams and saw me wake tired and annoyed and oh so bloody wet. I was second-guessing myself about whether doing this was the right thing to do – if by agreeing (OK, not even agreeing; let's remember the initial suggestion had been mine) that we meet for no-strings shenanigans I was basically starting myself back down a road I had travelled before with Thomas and had decided wasn't for me. But then, if I knew I wanted D/s in a relationship but didn't want a relationship, was it bad to want some no-strings fun with someone clearly filthy and trustworthy, with no baggage? Had I actually learned anything? Was this a terrible mistake? Was being frisky clouding my thinking?

In between all the, frankly, angsty thoughts that I couldn't quite push away, there was also a not-inconsiderable amount of anticipation building. The more I'd chatted to Adam, the more intrigued I'd become by him. I was still a bit pissed off by the fact that – thanks to Thomas and Charlotte's meddling – he'd known my sexual proclivities long before I had a whiff of his, almost an unfair advantage in our early conversations. But enough of what he had said had intrigued me, set me thinking and made me keen to see what he'd come up with and how he would lead me in a dynamic of dominance and submission.

I knew he didn't care for pain as much as any of the dominants I'd been with before – which was probably just as well, bearing in mind how I'd stubbed my toe in the office the day before and it had hurt so much I'd felt tears running down my cheeks. It would seem I was becoming a wuss. But he focused more on the satisfaction of humiliation, and the thought of that was intriguing and also a little nerve-wracking. I'd done lots of humiliating things before, most notably with Thomas and Charlotte, but they were in a wider context; the emphasis had still been more on pain. I knew I could cope with pain. What if the humiliation was too much? What if he annoyed me? What if I blushed? OK, it was definite I was going to blush, but what if it got too intense?

I tried to calm myself. If a hundred strikes of a wooden spoon directly between my legs was something I could withstand, surely I could cope with whatever he came up with, right? There was nothing he could say or do (or make me do – the thought slipped unbidden into my mind and threw up a whole new set of questions) that could be harder to cope with than that relentless pain, right? I wasn't so sure, mostly because I had no real understanding of what he would come up with. The unknown made me nervous and put me firmly on the back foot, which of course made me wet, which in turn made me grumpy. By the time he knocked on the door I was relieved – fifteen minutes longer and I might have over-thought myself into a headache.

When I opened the front door and saw him smile up at me from the front step my first thought was confusion. How had I not noticed his sharp jawline and how sexy his smile was? In the haze of fury at being stitched up on a blind date all I'd been aware of was his messy dark hair and a slightly smug air. The former was still apparent but there was no sign of the latter, well, not then anyway. Also, and forgive me for being a sucker for this kind of thing, he was wearing a suit. He wore it well.

We said hello, and I stepped back to let him in, suddenly feeling awkward. He walked past me and then stopped abruptly, unsure where to go next. I laughed, sounding high pitched to my own ears, and pointed down the corridor towards the living room, burbling nonsense to fill the now-slightly-awkward silence (well, it felt awkward to me).

'I haven't ever done this before, had someone round like this I mean. I'm not entirely sure what the etiquette of it is. Would you like a cup of tea, or coffee or –'

In hindsight I think it was probably best he moved when he did – otherwise I'd have gone through the entire beverage content of my kitchen one at a time. He moved so quickly I don't really know how I ended up with him pushed against me, his mouth on mine, the wall pressing into my back. I gasped in surprise, and he took advantage of me opening my mouth to insinuate his tongue, deepening the kiss.

He tasted of mint with a hint of coffee, presumably a lingering reminder of the lunch he'd just finished. As my surprise mellowed I began to kiss him back more aggressively. Suddenly our tongues were duelling and he was pushing me harder against the wall, holding me in place with his hips while his hands stroked up my arms, making me shiver a little, before softly touching the side of my face. He pushed a stray piece of hair behind my ear and I whimpered softly as his finger touched the shell-like curve. He smiled against my mouth and moved his hand back to do the same thing again, and I fought to control my reactions, trying to hold my own in the kiss, even while the meandering circles of his finger made my legs feel weak.

I don't know how long we stood there. Certainly by the time he broke off to look down at me for a moment, my nipples were hard in my bra and there was a flush in my cheeks. He stroked my hair gently and dropped a kiss onto the bridge of my nose.

'Are you ready? Are you sure you want to do this? If not, I'm perfectly happy to have tea.' He smiled at me, but there was mocking there. 'Or coffee. Milkshake if you have it, or –'

I shook my head firmly. 'I'm ready. I'm sure. Definitely.' I grinned at the ridiculousness of the conversation, realising how earnest I sounded.

He looked at me intently for a moment, as if he was checking for himself that what I was saying was the truth. Finally he nodded. 'Good. Remember what we said about safe words and limits. I'm going to go easy on you for now because this is our first time together, and I need to get to know your reactions, but if you need me to stop or slow down you know what to say?'

I nodded, sombre again and a little nervous. But then he leaned down again, his final 'Good' whispered against my bottom lip as he nipped it with his teeth before moving back to kiss me again.

Almost as soon as his mouth reconnected with mine the force of his kisses changed. It wasn't as if he had been a dainty kisser to start with, but now his mouth on mine was almost bruising with its intensity, pressing down as his tongue pushed its way in. He slid his hands round my arse, leaving my top half anchored firmly to the wall, while pushing my hips and waist into him.

I moved my arms up around his neck, urging him closer, but he tutted against my mouth, moving quickly again to grab both my wrists in one hand, pinning them above my head. I struggled for a minute, working to free them, but his hand was unmoving and I had a moment of realisation that he had me completely secure, followed quickly by a surge of lust. He wasn't much taller than me, but he had a wiry strength – there was no way I could get free without him letting me go. I shifted my wrists again, trying to move, and he was unyielding.

Suddenly his other hand wasn't stroking the side of my face tenderly. It was groping, pulling at my clothes, squeezing my breasts in turn, making me gasp, rolling my nipples between his fingers through my clothes. My brain froze in a moment of indecision, wondering whether to try harder to push him off, even while my body was curving into him, knowing how much the rough treatment was already turning me on. I smiled for a moment, amused that even now, after everything I had experienced, I still had that first instinct to push away, my mind rebelling against the truth my body, every fibre of my being, knew: that I wanted this. Craved it. I'd missed it. I couldn't wait to see where it was going to go.

I didn't have to wait long to find out.

Suddenly we were moving. He dragged me along the hallway, his hand still clasped tightly round my wrists. He stopped, momentarily, to check which room was the bedroom – *just as well I hadn't bought nibbles* – and then opened the door and pulled me inside. He let go of my wrists and sat down on the edge of the bed and I stood in front of him, unsure what to do next.

'Undress.'

Oh. OK. Well, not 'OK' really. Who wants to get naked this way the first time they sleep with someone? I know it sounds daft, but I figured that slipping my skirt off first would feel less embarrassing. Wearing a skirt was, and remains, a rarity for me, but he'd mentioned he liked hold-up stockings so I'd decided to make the effort. I stopped fiddling with the zip and finally let the skirt drop to the floor, the lining whispering as it slid down my legs and hit the ground. I'd been staring somewhere over his left shoulder while I did this, too embarrassed to actually look him in the face, but I couldn't help but sneak a peek at his expression, to see whether my black hold-ups met with his approval. I caught a glimpse of both his smile and the bulge in his trousers before I went back to staring at the wall – and the knowledge it was pleasing him made me brave. I began to undo the buttons of my blouse.

By the time my fingers, fumbling a little with a mixture of nerves and anticipation, had got to the bottom and I was ready to open my shirt my courage was beginning to falter. I haltingly opened the sides of my shirt and then, after a few seconds of silence, I slid my arms out and dropped it to the floor too.

I stood there in bra and knickers. I was probably about as covered as I would be at the beach, but felt much less comfortable or confident. I didn't want to make eye contact with him, but I wasn't sure what to do next. OK, I know what he wanted me to do next, I just wasn't sure I was able to do it. It felt like a pretty big leap.

His voice made me jump. 'Underwear too, come on.' I looked at him for a moment, and his gaze was reassuring, although his arms were folded, seemingly brooking no argument. 'Come on.'

I undid my bra first, freeing my breasts, blushing slightly as I unveiled my hard nipples to both our gazes – proof if any were needed that even while I was finding it difficult getting back into the submissive mindset (is it something you can just grow out of?), my body utterly approved of it. I felt my face get hot, making me worry about exactly how embarrassed I was looking. Beetroot red? Traffic-light red? Tomato red?

He leaned forward and his voice was kind, an acknowledgement of my struggle, but still no-nonsense. 'The knickers too. Come on. Stop prevaricating. I want to see your cunt. Although leave the hold-ups on. I love those.' He smiled at me. 'Dirty girl.'

That didn't help the blushing.

Slowly I hooked my fingers in the waistband of my knickers and slipped them down to my knees, unveiling myself to him before stepping out of them. I stood naked in front of him, the room silent for long seconds as he looked at me.

The embarrassment was beginning to get prickly. While I'm not too hung up on my looks, it takes a more confident and secure woman than me to feel anything other than shy and a bit embarrassed when I'm standing naked in front of the object of my desire, who is fully dressed and staring at me.

He shifted on the bed, slipping off his jacket and slowly and deliberately rolling up his sleeves. 'Turn around and face away from me.'

I should have felt relief – I could barely look him in the face as it was – but instead I felt the familiar internal struggle, exacerbated by an unexpected fury at the casual way he was now fiddling with something in his jacket pocket and not even looking at me, so certain of my obedience that he didn't even need to watch. Slowly I turned around, swallowing convulsively as I did so, fighting for self-control and to hide how much he was pushing my buttons.

He shifted from the bed, and suddenly I could smell his aftershave and feel his warmth and he was right behind me, leaning down a little so his breath was right next to my ear. I managed to fight off the urge to shiver, but I couldn't control my body enough to stop the goosebumps forming along my arms. My heart was pounding now, the mystery of what was going to happen next making me jittery, excited but nervous, the anticipation like those moments before a rollercoaster starts. I know it's a very niche rollercoaster, with more nakedness than would be usual, but stick with me.

He grabbed my wrists again, pulling them behind me, crossing them and holding them so they rested on my arse. As quickly as he was there he was gone, and I had a brief instinctive desire to move my hands, even though I knew – and he knew, too – I wasn't going to. I was going to wait, compliant in this position for whatever came next.

Very quickly, soft rope slid up my arms, looping over my naked shoulders. He tightened it and I couldn't move my arms back round even if I wanted to. He worked quickly, his fingers dexterous, looping the rope round my arms at intervals, above my elbows, at my forearms, tightening the loops, pulling my arms further backwards, pushing my breasts out, immobilising me in a way I'd never experienced before. It made my blood sing. When he got to my wrists he wrapped the rope tightly round itself over and over again, until my wrists felt like they were in the kind of cuffs that I was more used to. I tested my bonds, subtly, for me not him, and when I realised how completely secure I was I felt shocked at the warmth that flooded my belly. I'd never been tied tighter, and yet somehow the feeling was liberating. It made me wet.

There was a dull thump as he dropped the rest of the rope on the floor and walked in front of me, knocking me out of my reverie. I lowered my eyes, not ready to look at him yet, but he had other ideas. He put a finger under my chin and lifted it until I was staring at him. Neither of us spoke. He was grinning at me. It took serious self-control to resist the urge to kick him. I was still fantasising about doing just that when he dropped to his knees. The sudden movement confused me, and made me worry for a second that I actually had unwittingly lashed out. Then he picked up the rope and pulled it up between my legs. As he stood he winked at me, tugging the rope hard, which made it press against me. The two strands sat either side of my slit, pressing it together. He finished off by tying the remainder of the rope to the original loops round my shoulders. It was as though I was bloody gift-wrapped. The pressure of the rope between my legs, the eroticism, the powerlessness, all made me feel rather weak in the knees, but I was determined not to show weakness. I wasn't even going to give him a hint of my struggle, of how he was driving me to distraction, although I thought perhaps if his smile was anything to go by he might have had an idea.

He stood back, admiring the view – his ropework, my

body, perhaps a mixture of both – before walking behind me again. Suddenly not being able to see him and what he was doing made me nervous, and then his hands reached round, appearing in my field of view, roughly grabbing my breasts again. He groped and mauled them, his hands rough, his fingers pinching my nipples hard enough to make me wince, although I fought to breathe through my nose in a way that meant he didn't hear a tell-tale gasp. I knew it was pointless – he knew – but it still felt important to fight.

He leaned in, whispering in my ear that I was beautiful and brave but also extremely dirty for letting him do these things to me. I closed my eyes for a second, fighting for my composure before I turned to stare at him angrily. My fury made him laugh and his next words made me close my eyes again, this time in an embarrassed horror.

'Come on, Sophie, we both know it's true. If it isn't then the rope between your legs won't be wet when I check it, will it?'

Bastard.

He knew, I knew, that I was dripping. That the kissing, being incapacitated and humiliated had all helped raise the temperature between my legs. But suddenly I wanted to do everything in my power to stop him from finding out this inevitable fact.

His hand travelled down my body, skimming my sides, moving to my hips. I tried desperately to twist away, to close my legs, but my balance wasn't great and I stumbled a little. He grabbed hold of the rope anchoring my arms together, and pulled me back into position, hauling me upright, before his hands went back to my breasts. He leaned in again.

His voice in my ear wasn't loud, but it was stern and very serious. 'Stop messing about. Do what you're told or you'll regret it.'

I couldn't help myself. 'You've not told me to do anything. I'm not disobeying.'

I'm not sure what I expected but his laugh filled me with surprise and a surge of warmth. 'I was taking it as an implicit order that you keep your legs open when I am trying to get my hand in there.'

I swallowed again and nodded. I tried very hard to stay still as his hand went between my legs where, in paradoxical fashion, I was both yearning for him to be but didn't want him anywhere near. But, much to my frustration, he didn't touch my cunt. Instead he slid his fingers along the ropes on either side feeling, undoubtedly, how my arousal had made them damp. He laughed again, and I felt a surge of fury and humiliation. I'd never had someone embarrass me like this and it was incredibly frustrating – suddenly I was getting an understanding of his style of dominance, and it drove me to distraction.

He grabbed a handful of my hair and pulled me towards the bed. Again, the lack of movement of my arms paired with the rope between my legs made it difficult to balance but this time I didn't topple. I remained upright long enough for him to dump me face first onto the mattress, unable to cushion the fall with my pinioned arms.

He rolled me onto my side. It was marginally more comfortable, barring the rope digging into my hips, but it meant I could – finally – watch him undress. I stared at him greedily as he stripped, removing his clothes without embarrassment, with relish in fact. It made my position even more frustrating. I clenched my fists as well as I was able, wishing I could touch him, help, even possibly push him over.

Then he was standing in front of me, his cock pointing towards me with a pearl of pre-cum visible on the tip. Tempting. Oh so tempting. He was completely shaved, something I'd never experienced with a lover before, but something which I quickly realised I was going to enjoy.

He didn't speak, but as he moved closer to the bed I unthinkingly, desperately, opened my mouth, my yearning to taste him overcoming every other part of my brain. He didn't wait, and pushed quickly past my lips. I tried to suck him but he pulled out just as quickly before pushing forward again, not willing to even give me control of this single aspect, fucking my face instead, faster and rougher, grabbing my hair to pull me down on his cock until I could feel him pressing against my throat, making me gag and struggle to breathe.

As I spluttered a little, he pulled out for a moment, giving me, literally, breathing room to draw air into my lungs. His cock was in my eyeline, coated in a mixture of saliva and pre-cum, which he wiped across my face. I closed my eyes to try and hide it, but I felt my eyes fill with tears of shame and fury.

Suddenly I was moving – he was dragging me onto my front. I felt a surge of relief at the prospect of burying my face in the duvet, hiding my embarrassment, how much the humiliation was getting to me. I had a few seconds' respite as he moved behind me, although the tell-tale sound of the tear of a condom wrapper made it clear this was a temporary state. Then his hands were on my arse, spreading my cheeks and pulling on the rope, pressing it against my cunt in a way that made me bite down on my lip to suppress a whimper.

He climbed on top of me, pulling the rope aside. His legs were on the outside of mine, pressing them together, which made me feel even tighter than usual as he pressed his cock against my wetness. He pushed inside, leaning forward. His hands, either side of my head, took most of his weight but his body still pushed down on my bound arms, his breathing hard in my ears. He had overpowered me, immobilised me, and now he was using me, pushing deeper and deeper. It was intense, close, to the point of almost being claustrophobic. His body was barely moving above me to start with; instead it pinned me in place, another form of bondage to add to the rest.

I couldn't wait any longer. I shifted from underneath him, moving my hips in silent invitation for him to – please – fuck me. I couldn't bring myself to ask and he didn't answer, instead giving my arse a playful swat, which told me without words to stay still.

I remained unmoving, but it was torture. My arms were beginning to ache, and with his body pinning me down I could barely move anything. In a moment of clarity I was shocked to realise I was unconsciously curling and uncurling my toes – presumably because they were the only things that were free. Suddenly I was aware that my thighs were wet and I was desperate for him to start moving, although I knew there was no point trying to get him to before he was ready.

Finally he started fucking me, hard and rough, a pounding that meant that all of my attempts at silence were for naught, as I was suddenly moaning loudly, especially when he shifted slightly and suddenly the rope between my legs was rubbing against my clit. After all the teasing and anticipation my orgasm built quickly, and suddenly I was close to coming, feeling my thighs tremble with the onslaught. He realised the inevitable a couple of seconds later, but wouldn't even let me have control of this.

'Not yet, not until I say so,' he whispered in my ear.

I was trying to fend it off, to control myself, to please him, to show I could wait, but he was making it difficult; his relentless pace as he used me brought me ever closer to orgasming. His breath in my ear, the sound of him taking his pleasure, turned me on even more.

Finally, he took pity on me. 'Come now,' he said and I did, feeling him twitch and come inside me as my orgasm overcame me. My orgasm made my toes curl again but once I came down to earth I felt embarrassed and shy and a little grumpy: he had been able to control me so utterly.

His breath was still heavy from his own orgasm as he got up and began to untie me, and I felt oddly bereft at both being released and not having him on top of me. His face was endearingly serious as he told me he didn't want to keep me bound for too long for the first time. He checked my fingers for pins and needles and any arm stiffness from being tied for so long. I answered his questions honestly but in a kind of sleepy haze, the excitement of all we had done, paired with the power of my orgasm, meaning I was fit for little more than lying there staring at the beautiful criss-cross of rope marks on my arms, stroking my fingertips over them, loving how they felt. Finally, once I was untied and he had been assured that nothing was too painful or intense, he pulled me into a hug, pressing a kiss to my nose. I felt a surge of affection, still well and truly blissed out by all the feelings he had managed to elicit from my occasionally rebellious body.

It felt a bit incongruous, not least because I still knew so little about his everyday life. How did he take his tea? Which football team did he support? But somehow it felt like we fitted together very well.

We lay chatting for a long time afterwards. As I became slowly more coherent he asked me what I had enjoyed most, what I had found most difficult, the things I'd rather not do again and the things I definitely would. I'd never been with someone who'd discussed it in such depth in the immediate aftermath, and it felt so intimate. I could trust him with this stuff.

We stopped to kiss, often. He thanked me for being so obedient, pliant, fun. I grinned and blushed and tried not to look him in the eye as he discussed the ruder things. Suddenly, in spite of myself, I started to think more fondly of Thomas's and Charlotte's cack-handed matchmaking.

We'd agreed he wouldn't stay over, but he didn't leave until 2 a.m., and only then because we both had early starts the following day and he'd have had to drive across the city in rush hour. We never did eat the cookies. I sent him home with most of them in a little Tupperware container, feeling a bit silly as I handed it over, but at the same time wanting him to have the biscuits I'd baked for him. The following day he messaged me a picture of a cookie sitting next to his mug of tea at work. It made me smile. I emailed a response. Suddenly we were chatting again.

Chapter Three

I knew even before he'd left that night that I wanted to see him again. I know! So much for all my 'no strings, this is just fun' stuff. What can I say? I liked him. He was funny, self-deprecating and good to talk to. In between sexual shenanigans we lay in the dark chatting about politics and TV, work stuff and films. It made me a little grumpy to concede it, and I still didn't approve of their tactics in the least, but Charlotte and Thomas had found exactly the kind of guy I'd like to date.

That biscuit-related message was the first of many that he sent over the next few weeks, and I was very happy indeed to reply. We chatted about lots of different things – from stories I was working on to issues he was having with a colleague at work – and he began to nip over after work during the week if we were both free. We'd leap on each other as soon as he came through the door, kissing urgently, pulling at each other's clothes, desperate to sate our sexual appetites on each other. It was wonderful, primal, so much bloody fun. We'd drink tea and chat about nothing in particular afterwards, and it was relaxing and easy and not awkward. I came to look forward to his visits, and was beginning to realise that he was pretty much my ideal kinky boyfriend material.

Except, of course, we'd kind of already agreed we

weren't going to date, agreed that this was to be a no-strings sort of thing. Balls.

Of course, on the plus side, this whole 'we weren't going to date' thing made for some full and frank discussions of the kind that might have been slightly more awkward with a man you were considering might be a permanent relationship fixture. Which is how he ended up breaking into my house to jump me as I slept.

OK, I'm over-egging that a little. But not much.

We were discussing long-standing fantasies. Things we'd always wanted to try but which, for one reason or another, hadn't been able to do. I was less experienced than him, particularly in D/s terms, so my list was quite a bit longer than his, and as we lay in bed chatting about it, him running his fingertips up and down my arm, he seemed particularly interested in my yearning to be overpowered in my sleep – to wake up to someone pinning me down and hurting me, fucking me.

As ever, this is all about the fantasy. I am a security-minded person. My window locks were always locked, and I wasn't yearning to be burgled or raped and attacked in my own home by a stranger. It needed to be someone I trusted, someone I wanted to fuck, within the previously agreed (but admittedly rough D/s style) boundaries, but I loved the idea of being taken by surprise.

We talked about it for a long while, and even the chat made me wet. I spoke haltingly, my voice quiet – even with my general openness about fantasies, and knowing that Adam knew the context in which we would be operating, it still felt pretty taboo talking about wanting to be woken up by someone fucking me. Adam was louder, more confident, and also clearly enjoying the chat, if his erection pressing into my arse as he whispered in my ear was anything to go by. As he asked more questions and I stumbled a little answering them, I realised he was revelling in my embarrassment and awkwardness, enjoying the little humiliations of discussing this, knowing how wet it was making me. Adam's different style of dominance was taking a little getting used to, and seemed to put me on the back foot even more than my previous experiences. While he wasn't averse to inflicting some nipple pinching or a spanking in the right mood, his dominance was as much psychological – about words and actions rather than pain. It consistently boggled my mind how he could get me into a deeply submissive and compliant mindset without the pain that had so far formed such a key part of my D/s experiences.

By the time we had finished discussing it and he had told me how it could work he had slipped his hand between my legs and was telling me how filthy I was for getting off on the idea of it. There was even a kind of plan.

I didn't have a spare key. If I had the whole thing would have been much easier. As it was, the slight danger of it meant it took me a while to fall asleep the night before I knew it was to happen.

We'd agreed that I would put my front-door key in an envelope inside my paper recycling bin, which sat next to my front door. Even if someone did come up to my front door to rummage through the cereal boxes and old newspapers, the hope was that an old junk-mail envelope, seemingly stuck to the inside by a stray piece of tape, would be overlooked. It would be a pretty big leap to assume it would contain a key that would open my front door – at least that's what I told myself as I lay in bed trying to get to sleep after I'd snuck out into the dark and deserted street at midnight to stick it in place.

It took a long time to go to sleep. I was wearing a slightly sexier pair of knickers than I normally would have – my fashion choices for bed tended to be nothing at all or fleecy pyjamas depending on the weather, and we were definitely still in the PJ comfort side of the year, although I'd decided against them just this once. I couldn't get comfortable, and I was nervous about the key being outside (even though I knew it would be fine and even if anyone had seen me out there all they had seen was my putting some old newspapers in the recycling) and about what Adam would do to me when he got in. He'd asked me not to orgasm before bed, and while part of me chafed at the edict, it seemed churlish to quibble when he had agreed to fulfil such a long-held fantasy. But my body was used to falling asleep in a post-orgasm haze most nights so it made it even harder to drop off. I sat watching the luminous dial of the clock change, my brain ticking away, my imagination and nerves getting ever more fanciful, and me getting ever more grumpy. I wasn't going to fall asleep like this.

I had an itchy nose, or there was something on my face. I tried to move my arm from under the duvet to swat whatever it was away but it seemed to be tangled up. I struggled for a minute before I sleepily turned my face towards the pillow instead. But moving felt difficult, like wading through treacle.

Suddenly I was awake with a start, my heart pounding as I realised there was someone lying on the bed with me, on top of the duvet, their body partially over mine, making it difficult to move from under the covers. I knew it was him. I was sure it was him. It smelt like him, I think, like the familiar smell of his aftershave. I think. But I couldn't see his face, and I was nervous, in need of reassurance. What if it wasn't him? What if someone else saw me sticking the envelope to the side of the box? What if it was the guy from over the road who took a parcel in for me once? Or a random teenage boy walking home late at night who'd seen my furtive rummaging? I knew my imagination and nerves were running away with me, but I couldn't see him. I needed to be sure. I opened my mouth to say his name before my sleep-dulled brain realised I couldn't because there was a hand clasped over my mouth. I was confused. The bedroom was lit with an early-morning glow. I guessed it must be 6 or 7 a.m. After all my worries about being unable to sleep I seemed to have dropped off just fine. Too well, in fact. If I'd just been able to sneak a peek at his face to be sure I'd have been enjoying it much more. Instead there was a tinge of fear, of danger. What if it wasn't him? Could I be sure?

I shifted on the bed, trying to struggle from within my cocoon, to shift myself round, to catch a glimpse of him, just long enough to know for definite. He pushed his weight down further, and I harrumphed into his hand, grumbling my concerns, a whimper in my throat trying to explain something, anything, just to get him to respond. If he spoke I'd have known it was him and then I would have been OK. My nostrils filled with the smell of leather as his gloved hand tightened against my mouth, pressing hard against my lips, and suddenly his voice was whispering a 'sssssshhhhhh' in my ear. Was it an echo of the man I lay here with days ago discussing how hot this was, or someone else completely? The longer we lay there, the more certain I was it was the former not the latter, but even with just five per cent uncertainty my stomach cramped with a little fear.

He moved, but his hand was still tight round my mouth. I tried to press my teeth into his palm but there was no room for manoeuvre, even if I had been able to nip hard enough to hurt him through his glove. I waited for what was to happen next, my heart beating loudly in my ears. There was a sudden rush of cold air as the duvet was pulled away. I got goosebumps at the abrupt change in temperature, and grabbed to pull it back, for the safety and warmth. He levered me onto my back and pushed harder against my mouth in warning. I remained still, swallowing convulsively, finally getting my chance to look him in the eyes. It was him. While I knew that rationally it had to be him, the relief of knowing for sure was like a headrush. But the nerves didn't dissipate. His eyes were assessing me, and I'd never felt more, well, naked. I tried to still my breathing so my breasts didn't bounce quite as obviously as he stared at me, and I waited to see what would happen next, where this was going to go.

He didn't speak, but once more his palm pressed firmly against my mouth in warning before he loosened his grip just a little. His hand stayed there, though, while the other began to explore my body, his touch neither tender nor friendly. He was pawing at me, groping my breasts. His eyes filled with lust, and suddenly I was wishing I'd gone for my fleecy pyjamas after all. He lifted my hip and slid his hand underneath to grab a handful of my arse and I took the opportunity to shuffle across the bed a little, trying to avoid the worst of his punishing grip, deciding this was my best opportunity to struggle.

Big mistake. His hand tightened against my mouth again and the look in his eyes was enough to stop me, intense enough to make me wary. I was suddenly nervous that I'd made him angry, and cursed my inner rebellion. His other hand was no longer mauling my arse, but I'll be honest, that didn't feel exactly like a victory. Fear cramped my stomach as I considered what would happen next.

He leaned over me, his face looming close to mine, and I expected him to tell me off, use stern words, give me a warning. What I was not expecting was for his other hand to pinch my nose closed. I panicked.

We'd talked about breath play before. It's something I'd read about, but not something I'd ever done. I knew he liked it, he knew I was curious to try it, we had discussed how it would work, how he would keep me safe, how he could read the signs of when it was too much or not enough. In our nuzzled-together post-coital chats it had sounded dark but hot, something I could cope with, but now it was happening, my brain broke a little.

I felt fear. I tried to quell the rising panic, but my chest tightened as my lungs fought to take in more air. My heart raced as I struggled. His hands were firm, still, and his expression was implacable, his whole stance calm as every part of my body filled with fear and panic. A hysterical half thought bubbled up from my mind – he had power over everything, in this moment he controlled whether I could breathe. It shocked me, I'd never felt so controlled, but there was no time to think rationally about it. Finally he let go. It seemed like it had been an eternity, but it was probably just a few seconds. I sucked deep breaths in through my nose, the sound loud in the room.

For long moments we just stared at each other. I was wary; the look on his face was stern, but I knew he was checking my reaction, making sure that I was OK. He still didn't say anything, but suddenly he leaned down and gently kissed my forehead. His hand was still clasped over my mouth and the tenderness paired with the threat of violence was an odd thing to experience, but it made me melt. I tried to smile at him with my watery eyes. He waited a moment longer, before seeing whatever it was that he wanted to see, and finally released me.

The relief I felt didn't last long. He reached down to the floor to pick something up. I couldn't quite see what it was, but it seemed to be deliberately out of my sightline. How had he been able to unpack without me noticing?

He brought up a ball gag and pressed the large red bulb of it to my mouth. I swallowed, trying to minimise the saliva that I knew the gag would end up collecting, but then opened my mouth compliantly as he pushed it inside. I don't think I even glared at him, such was the level of my obedience. It would appear breath play and sleepiness made for an especially submissive Soph. He lifted my head up gently so he could fasten the leather straps of the gag without pulling my hair too much, and I smiled to myself at the paradox of a man who enjoyed being able to hurt me – but only wanted to do so by design rather than accident.

He reached down again. I considered taking a peek to see exactly what he'd put on the floor by my bed. I was agog at how long he must have been here while I slept. So much for me being a pretty light sleeper. Was I in a really deep sleep or did he have more experience of creeping into women's houses in the early hours of the morning than I first anticipated? I didn't dare move to look, though – he already seemed to be in a fiendish mood and even I have a basic instinct for self-preservation in such situations. Mostly.

This time it was a short length of rope. He grabbed my wrists and quickly wrapped them with the soft cotton. It wasn't his prettiest rope tie, but it was secure and tight. He attached the end to the headboard and suddenly I was extremely exposed in my little lace knickers. He was looking down at me and smiling, but his smile was wolfish, a 'now I have you where I want you' look. I was nervous, although I felt myself getting wetter; the knowledge it wouldn't be too long before he realised that too made me blush.

He leaned down again and picked something up, then was back at the headboard. He pressed a small bell into my hand, the kind you might have on a cat's collar or something similar. This was my safety net; if I dropped it, he would stop, taking it in lieu of a safe word since I was unable to speak. I clasped my hand around it tightly, clinging on for dear life, although I don't know if that was because I wanted to be ready to drop it – or was afraid that I might do so accidentally. Ah, the paradoxes of submission – and my contrary mind.

Adam climbed onto the bed, straddling my body. He unzipped and pulled out his hard cock, resting it between my breasts, just inches from my mouth (although that was somewhat academic with the gag wedged tightly between my lips).

I realised a second too late that he'd picked something else up. There was no time to struggle, nowhere to go even if I could. The sunlight glinted on the chain as it dropped from his hand. It was a set of nipple clamps. He took his time attaching them to my breasts, enjoying my wary expression, my attempts to swallow nervously round the gag as my eyes looked anxiously at the fierce-looking metal clasps. He took the opportunity to grope my breasts, pinching my nipples, rolling them between his fingers, laughing softly at my flush of shame at how erect they were from the twisted scenario playing out between us. When he finally attached the clamps, the pain was less than I feared, but the whole experience of having had them put on had been intense. It was an odd feeling – he wasn't into inflicting pain in the sadistic way that James had been, but he seemed to get off on the embarrassment I experienced at how aroused the pain made me. It was a whole different kind of head fuck and I couldn't process it – although, let's face it, it's a miracle any of this made sense before my first cup of coffee of the day.

Once he had attached the clamps – and given one a firm tug to be sure they were secure (he got a glare then) – he lay down next to me on the bed. We must have made an odd picture, him dressed in jeans and a dark woollen jumper looking for the most part like he was about ready for a trip out for morning Starbucks, lying on his side with his head resting on one hand, staring at me. Next to him I was mostly naked, blushing, with bed head, a little drool round the mouth and incredibly erect nipples. The ridiculousness of it made me smile, even while I was warily watching him to see what happened next.

Slowly, languidly, he started playing with my body. He wasn't as rough as before, more teasing and meandering with his touch, enjoying watching me shiver at the feeling of his leather-covered fingertips moving along my skin, watching the goosebumps rise on my body, smiling when I sucked air in deeply through my nose and tried to regulate my breathing as he wrung those little reactions from me. He grazed my thighs, ran a finger along the chain between my breasts, laughing softly at my look of nervousness before just gently tugging it. He stroked my hair off my face, chuckling softly as I blushed when he noticed the drool pooling in the corner of my mouth because of the gag. He was like a child with a new toy, and all I could do was lie there and take it, clutching the bell and waiting for what he would do next.

After several stray strokes of my thighs, my hips and the scalloped edge of my knickers, finally he put a hand between my legs, over the lace. I knew I was going to be wet and warm; despite the chill in the room this whole experience had left me flushed and hot. He pressed his palm against my cunt, his eyes looking into mine as he did so, and his smile – bordering on the smug – and his obvious amusement at how embarrassed I was made me harrumph behind my gag. In a surge of annoyance I closed my legs and tried to shuffle my lower body away, glaring at him as I lifted my hips for purchase. He slapped my thigh – hard enough that I noticed a red hand imprint for a second afterwards. His voice sounded unreal, far away. It was the first thing he'd said since I woke up.

'Behave.'

I looked at him, feeling my nostrils flare, feeling the fury and rebellion rise, knowing that I was fighting not just him but the part of me that was clearly aroused by this, enjoying every kinky minute of it.

He pinched my inner thigh, a hard, painful pinch of warning. I whimpered quietly. He looked at me, not quite sure yet what my reaction would be, seemingly ready to decide his course of action depending on what happened next. Annoyingly, I knew exactly what my reaction would be, it was inevitable, even while part of me baulked against it. I glared at him, trying to swallow some of the drool pooling behind my gag. And then I looked away, unwilling to see his look of victory up close – he really could be so fucking smug – as slowly I opened my legs.

His hand went back to my knickers, stroking up and down, making the material wetter. He was still playing. There was no time limit to this, and he enjoyed teasing. Sometimes he placed a little pressure on my clit and I moaned through the gag. The intensity of this all paired with the lack of orgasm before bed the previous night had left me a ball of desperate nerve endings. I was impatient but nervous, desperate to continue but worried about what that meant. I wanted to make him proud, make him happy, kick him off the bed, come.

After a while he seemed to decide that he'd made my knickers wet enough. He moved from his position next to me on the bed, kneeling instead between my legs where – I knew – he had a great view of the shiny dampness of my once-posh and now incredibly slutty-looking undies. I closed my eyes again. It just made it a little less embarrassing.

He lifted my knees and pushed them back to my chest. Even with my underwear on I felt incredibly exposed; even with my eyes closed I could sense his gaze looking between my legs. I felt him move on the bed, his hands still holding me up and open, his fingers pinching a little as I lay immobilised. He licked my thigh just at the edge of my knickers. I shivered. He moved to the other thigh and did the same thing again, and this time I fought to control my reactions. I was swimming against the tide of sensation, though. He moved and rested his mouth just centimetres from my cunt, his breath warm and steady – much steadier than mine, I realised with frustration – against me.

At last. One long lick, from the bottom to the top of my cunt. Over the knickers, so it shouldn't have felt as intense as it did, but fuck it really did. It made my thighs shake with the sensation of it. Too much teasing makes for an overwrought Sophie it would seem. He was back to playing, licking me over and over again, but still over the sodding (and sopping) knickers. It took all my self-control (and not a little bit of self-preservation) to resist the urge to kick him in the shoulder, so desperate was I to feel his tongue directly on me. I raised my hips in eager invitation, silently – but admittedly unsubtly – imploring him to take more of me in his mouth. All to no avail. He looked up at me, the gleam in his eye showing as much as the bulge at his groin that he was enjoying himself. Git.

I lost track of how long I had been on the edge of desperation. He placed his hands on the waistband of my knickers and I gratefully, hastily, lifted myself up so he could pull them down my legs and off. He chucked them aside and his mouth was back on me, no teasing now, he was practically drinking me as he pushed his tongue inside me, moving his face from side to side so his nose pushed against my clit until I whimpered desperately behind the gag. Then he took my clit in his mouth directly and began sucking on it, closing his lips tightly around it, flicking his tongue over it, again and again and again until my long-awaited orgasm consumed me, lifting me off the bed in convulsions, my cries muffled by the gag in a way that probably worked out for the best where my neighbours were concerned.

It was intense. The whole experience had been intense. There wasn't time to recover yet, though. As my breathing began to slow he stood up and stripped, grabbing a condom from the pocket of his jeans before throwing them, along with the gloves and his clothes, on the floor. Stopping briefly to put it on, he came back to the bed and pushed himself deeply inside me, even as I was still throbbing with the aftermath of my orgasm.

He lay down so most of his weight was on top of me, his face close to mine, smiling, even while he took his pleasure from my body, moving his full length in and out of me slowly, pushing himself deep enough that his pelvis hit my clit, making me whimper again. Every movement brushed against the nipple clamps, and the constant movement made my nipples ache in a way that I found distracting – the mixture of pain and pleasure and being tied down somehow tamped down my occasional rebellions, leaving me feeling a desperate yearning to please him, to give him – admittedly in a very different way – the kind of pleasure he had just given me. In that moment I would have done or endured anything he wanted me to, and the best way of showing him that felt like bucking my hips in inviting fashion.

We kept the rhythm moving, as he reached behind my head to remove the gag. I desperately swallowed the worst of my drool as he pulled it out, laughing as he apologised at accidentally pulling my hair as he undid the buckle. He raised an eyebrow and I instantly felt a bit chagrined.

'Sorry, I just found it a bit funny. Torturing my nipples is fine, but accidental hair-pulling needs an apology.'

'There's no excuse for impoliteness,' he said, grabbing a handful of hair and pulling it much harder than he'd done by accident a moment before. I laughed again, but it was swallowed into a kiss as he moved his mouth over mine. I smiled against his mouth and began reciprocating eagerly, although the taste of myself on his lips made me blush again – it was as if his aim in life was to leave me constantly embarrassed and wet.

As we kissed he fucked me harder, pulling out slowly but pushing back in with a force that left me gasping into his mouth. After a few moments he lifted his head away from me and looked straight into my eyes, his expression suddenly sombre. Keeping most of his weight on one hand, he placed the other around my throat.

It was an entirely involuntary reaction, but my entire

body went stiff. Just having his fingers resting there made me nervous. I closed my eyes, trying to hide my nerves, but his voice was firm.

'Look at me.'

It took a couple of deep, steadying breaths before I could open my eyes and meet his gaze. When I did his look was serious, but calm.

'Do you trust me?'

I'd repeatedly let him tie me up and given him the key to my flat and an open invitation to come round and assault me in my sleep. If the answer was 'no' I was clearly an idiot, but even so, saying it aloud felt like a big step.

'Yes, I trust you,' I said, my voice quiet and a little shy, because I did, and part of me was wondering how the fuck that could be when I had only met him so relatively recently.

He nodded, and put pressure on my throat, making it hard for me to breathe. I gasped, my breathing rasping as I tried to drag air into my lungs, watching him watching me, making sure that I was OK. As he let go, again after a couple of seconds, I felt a surge of adrenaline, and surprise at how this turned me on, and it really had, if my involuntary hip bucking underneath him as he choked me was anything to go by.

We kept fucking, alternating between leisurely bucking and moments when he grabbed me by the throat. He held my neck for longer as I began to get used to it, but still never for more than a few seconds at a time. I loved the feeling of it – the powerlessness, the restriction, paired with the lustful, greedy look he would get on his face and the way he would fuck me harder, pounding me till it was

61

almost hurting but at the same time getting me closer to a second orgasm. Finally he choked me one last time – with the most pressure and for the longest period so far – as my orgasm hit again. My back arched with the force of it and he released his grip round my throat, so I could take in a deep, dizzying lungful of air as I came. My frenzied movements seemed to push him over the edge, with him coming inside me a few short seconds afterwards, moaning out his own pleasure. Thankfully he didn't collapse onto the clamps afterwards, instead lying down carefully next to me again, looking slightly more mussed himself now.

We were both still breathing heavily as he untied my hands and carefully removed the nipple clamps, rubbing feeling gently back into my aching nipples as they began to tingle painfully back into life.

Finally, he leaned down the bed and grabbed the duvet, covering us both up and enveloping me in a cuddle. We chatted about how things had gone and how I had found being choked, and then I dozed off, waking only to the smell of bacon and freshly brewed coffee – to top it all off Adam had brought breakfast in his bag of supplies.

As fantasies go the reality was pretty bloody amazing. It made me suddenly desperate to think about all the other things I wanted to try, happy I had a partner in crime I could do them with. Although not *that* way, because obviously we weren't going to be dating. We'd decided. Obviously.

Fuck. Who was I kidding?

Chapter Four

The next few weeks passed in a further flurry of emails and texts messages, mixed with some truly memorable late-night phone conversations – and an increasing number of visits. Adam would come round, we would do scandalous things to each other and then, once we were both exhausted and sated, he would do the long journey home to minimise faff for his early starts to work.

But then slowly things began to change. He still came round of an evening, but we would eat together. He took me out for a leisurely curry one night. We jumped each other afterwards (albeit tentatively – we'd eaten a *lot* of curry) but spending time together where we weren't having sex was beginning to be as fun as the filthy things we got up to between the sheets. And on my sofa. In the shower. You know what I mean. Then he came round so I could cook him lamb tagine – something he'd always been intrigued to try but hadn't had the chance to. It took ages, so we ate late and it just seemed to make sense for him to stay over. I suggested it, aiming for a casualness I wasn't sure I could quite pull off, and he agreed, similarly casually. And then we just grinned at each other like idiots for a little while, until we dozed off.

Suddenly I was thinking about our lively debates about politics or discussion about the best Bond film of all time as much as the way he'd tied me to the bed and licked me until I whimpered the morning after we'd spent a night together (although, obviously, that was bloody amazing too).

He began to visit for weekends, often arriving late on Friday night so we could spend all of Saturday together before either working or fulfilling other social commitments on the Sundays. It was a weird middle-ground: we weren't dating, and it's not as if I've ever been a 'joined at the hip, must do everything together' kind of girlfriend anyway, but I began to look forward to our weekend routine, while trying my very best to not overthink it and instead just enjoy it for what it was.

Of course, as ever, not knowing exactly what our relationship was made me feel a little unsure of myself at times, not least when he mentioned, in passing, that he'd slept with Charlotte a few times.

We were discussing hotels when he mentioned it. Not in an inappropriate way – one of the lovely things about Adam was the fact that when he wasn't being incredibly rude he was very gentlemanly. We were talking about going to see a gig and, as he began to realise how for me the attraction of seeing any band on a big arena tour has to be offset by exactly how difficult it is to get home afterwards, he suggested trying to find a nearby hotel. We Googled to find what was available and, as he leaned over to see what had come top of the list, he dropped the bombshell.

'Nah, not that one. Charlie and I stayed there once, it was a total dive.'

I was confused. Was I supposed to know who that was? Had I not been listening when he'd told me about his friend? 'Charlie? Who's Charlie? Were you at another gig?'

64

'Definitely not a gig, but there was a performance element.' He smiled a bit at the memory. 'Charlie. Charlotte, Charlie. It was a fetish club night.'

I hoped my eyes weren't cartoonishly wide, but it took a moment for the penny to drop.

'Thomas's Charlotte?' He didn't call her 'Charlie'. In fact I hadn't heard anyone else call her that but Adam.

'Yeah, that Charlie.' He held his hands up. 'But she wasn't seeing Thomas then. It was a casual thing for both of us. It only happened a few times.' He looked at my face, and I dread to think what he saw there, but he clarified some more. 'And it hasn't happened for ages.'

I didn't know what to say. I know this is unreasonable, bearing in mind I too had seen Charlotte naked, but I felt a horrible feeling in the pit of my stomach that I was pretty sure was jealousy. He was looking at me worriedly. 'Soph, I'm sorry, I thought she'd mentioned it.'

His concern was sweet, seemingly heartfelt, and reassured me that he wasn't some kind of player. I hoped. I smiled and tried to stop overthinking things. 'It's OK. I didn't know, but it's not my business anyway really.' The silence lengthened and I suddenly thought through the rest of his sentence and burst out laughing. 'Hold on, a fetish party? I don't even know what that is. I'm like the BDSM country mouse visiting the town mouse hanging out with you.'

He grinned and pulled me into a cuddle. 'Stick with me, little mouse. I'm sure I can open you up to all kinds of new experiences.'

He wasn't kidding.

Adam was definitely broadening my sexual horizons.

There didn't seem to be many things he hadn't tried or didn't want to try. He was very experimental and creative, and his ability to make me blush at his suggestions for things we could do became legendary.

I didn't feel inadequate in our rude chats. I was more than happy holding my own in a smutty conversation and he often commented on how refreshing he found it to be able to chat so openly about sex. But I wanted to do more; I wanted to show him that he wasn't the only one with an imagination. It took a little preparation but within a week or so I had ideas for a couple of erotic surprises, thanks to some well-thought-out internet shopping.

As we were a pair of news nerds we increasingly found ourselves on a Saturday morning, after some early morning fun, sat on the comfy sofa in a local cafe, drinking coffee, eating pastries and swapping sections of the broadsheets.

On one such Saturday I put my plan into action. We'd booked tickets for an early showing at the cinema, and were enjoying killing time reading out stories we found interesting and mocking each other's choice of newspaper.

I was incredibly nervous when I excused myself to go to the bathroom. He didn't notice, though, too wrapped up in the cricket reports from the previous day's test.

When I returned a few minutes later I had a small box in my hand. It had a neat ribbon tied round it, and a little note tucked under the bow – if there was one thing playing with Adam had taught me, it was that details mattered.

I popped the box onto his lap and smiled at him as he looked up at me, slightly confused.

'What's this?' he asked. 'It's not my birthday.'

I knew when his birthday was. He'd casually mentioned it in passing a few weeks before and I'd added it to my online calendar the following day. I wasn't sure if it sounded a bit too keen to admit that, though, so I ignored it.

'You should open it.' I was blushing. For a change.

Still bemused, he slipped the ribbon off and removed the lid. He lifted out a small plastic object with a couple of buttons on it; it looked not unlike a garage door opener or some such gadget. He clearly was none the wiser. I felt a surge of smugness. I'd obviously stumped him.

It didn't stop my voice sounding a little husky with embarrassment when I spoke, though. 'You should read the note.'

He unfolded the piece of paper and read the words I'd written on it in neat blue handwriting.

I think we both know you have the ability to push my buttons in all the fun ways. Now you can do so literally. You're holding the remote control to a vibrating egg. I'm sure you can guess where it is right now. The buttons will turn the vibrations on and off and vary the speed. Do you want to play?

His face lit up like an overexcited kid on Christmas morning and I grinned to myself, knowing that the gadget element would appeal to him.

His whisper was part wonder, part awareness that there were folk around us who neither of us wanted to be part of our game. 'This is brilliant. You're brilliant. I've never even heard of this, much less used one.'

He folded the note neatly into the box with the ribbon,

before sliding it back into my handbag. He put the remote control in his pocket.

It didn't take him long to find the on switch. I'd reached for my coffee and I almost threw it over myself as I suddenly felt the vibrations deep inside me. I looked at him and he grinned.

He left it on and gradually increased the speed. I tried to read my paper but it was impossible. I couldn't concentrate on anything, and my hand was still shaking, which made lifting my mug a dangerous sport.

I leaned over, resting my head on his shoulder as if reading his paper with him but the truth was I was just hanging on for dear life. There was no way I would orgasm like this in public – at least I hoped there wasn't – but I was becoming increasingly wet and embarrassed. I cursed myself for coming up with such a daft idea. I suddenly had *When Harry Met Sally* flashbacks. And no one wants that.

As my fingernails dug into his arm, suddenly it all stopped. I realised how tense I had been as I finally relaxed, returning to my side of the sofa. I was breathing hard, my chest rising and falling. Thankfully there wasn't anyone sitting too close. They might have been worried I was having an asthma attack.

He pulled his hand out of his pocket to turn the page of his paper and started chatting to me as if nothing was any different. I slowly returned to normal and began to relax as we finished our drinks.

We got up and headed for the exit. When he held the door open for me I didn't realise his hand was in his pocket. As I exited to the sunny pavement I felt a pulse in my cunt and I almost stumbled as I let out a short, high-pitched squeak. No one seemed to notice but he laughed as he walked out behind me, musing at how much fun this was going to be. His power-crazy look made me laugh, although I was wondering exactly how I was going to sit through a film and focus. Thank goodness we'd gone for a popcorn flick with lots of explosions rather than anything too highbrow.

I received a couple more surprises as we walked to the cinema, but he mostly left me alone. He thanked me for handing him such control, but warned that he wasn't going to be all that responsible with it, in case I hadn't already guessed.

We took our seats. I get irate at the amount of adverts they show before a film at the best of times, but with Adam using the time to torture me, I was more desperate for the trailers to start than ever. He pressed all the buttons and asked me what all the different settings were doing to me – constant vibrations, pulses, etc. I explained as best I could, whispering through gritted teeth, as he cycled through the programmes.

I think it would have been easier to focus if he had just left the toy vibrating but he spent the next two hours tormenting me. He made sure to change the setting before I got used to what I was feeling, driving me crazy and causing me to hold on to him once again.

At one point, when the explosions were especially loud so the few people in the cinema sitting near us couldn't possibly overhear, he leaned in to whisper in my ear, to ask if I was wet. I hid my face in the crook of my arm as I nodded.

He put his hand on my inner thigh and moved it

upwards – thank goodness Saturday-morning cinema-goers tend to flock to more family-friendly films than we had so there was no one in our row. He slowly moved his little finger up and down the seam of my jeans and told me that he could actually feel the vibrations.

It was at that point I kicked him in the shin. I was beyond caring if it would get me into trouble, although he later admitted he probably deserved my admonishment. He removed his hand and put it over my shoulders, keeping the remote in his other hand and making sure I never settled. The film pretty much passed me by – he later bought it for me on DVD as a gift – and by the time it finished I only had one thing on my mind, and it wasn't the mark-ups on over-priced cinema popcorn. Finally, the lights went up. He was grinning at me.

'So. What do you want to do next?'

I couldn't speak for a minute. What on earth did he think I wanted to do?

'Lunch?' He was having so much fun. I wasn't sure if I found him endearing or annoying. The throbbing between my legs wasn't helping me decide.

In the end I thought politeness might work more in my favour.

'Can we go home? Please?'

He stroked my arm with his fingertips and I shivered. There was no way I was going to manage eating lunch without throwing it all over the place. After long, desperate seconds he took pity on me.

'Of course we can.'

He left the egg on a constant setting all the way home but it still pulsed as I walked and I still didn't seem to be able to ignore it, not least because the weighted egg shifted inside me as I moved, sparking sharp waves of pleasure.

As we got back to my flat I felt him turn it off for the first time in hours. I became aware of how wet I was and wondered if I'd get the chance to sort myself out and change my underwear before he decided to do anything fiendish with me. Not a chance. Definitely optimistic.

As soon as we entered the living room he was behind me. His hands wrapped around my body, groping my breasts as his mouth found my neck and shoulder, kissing and gently biting me. It was as though he had been waiting for the moment we closed the door behind us and had privacy. Suddenly I realised I had inadvertently been teasing him for as long as he had been teasing me.

He unbuttoned my jeans, shifting them down my hips and putting his hand between my legs.

He chuckled softly. 'Your knickers are soaking.'

I tried to press my thighs together but he gave them a quick slap so I left them open. He pushed me forward, bending me over the arm of my sofa, pulling my knickers down to join my jeans around my thighs.

He reached forward and took hold of the thin plastic cord protruding from my cunt and pulled it. I gasped as the egg popped out into his hand.

Within seconds I was gasping again. I hadn't heard him unzip himself or the tell-tale sound of the condom wrapper being pulled open, but without warning he had pushed himself all the way inside me. I was so wet that he slid in easily but I cried out in surprise, my fingernails digging into the cushion as he began to move.

His hand moved to my mouth, pressing something to

my lips. It took a second to click, but it was the egg that had spent so long inside me. I clenched my teeth shut.

For a moment he stilled, then he pulled my hair in warning. I opened my lips, taking the wet toy into my mouth, tasting myself on it.

He kept fucking me hard and it wasn't too long before I felt him go stiff as his orgasm hit him. His breathing was heavy as he moved to dispose of the condom. When he returned he held his hand out under my face and I opened my mouth, letting the egg fall into his outstretched palm.

He helped me into a sitting position on the sofa and pulled my legs forward and open as he knelt on the floor in front of me. Within seconds he was licking me. As with the sex, there was no preamble, no teasing, just a relentless, firm pressure on my clit as he licked and sucked it. I felt his fingers between my legs and then I felt him push the toy back inside me.

He turned it on and I bucked my hips up, grinding myself against his face as he continued to focus on my clit. He put it on the fastest setting and flicked his tongue over me again and again. My hands were in his hair and I was moaning loudly. I was lost.

'Please may I come?' I groaned. I know. It wasn't something I made a habit of asking without being explicitly told to, but I wasn't risking everything stopping for any reason.

He nodded his permission as he kept licking. I thrust upwards again and kept hold of his hair. It felt as though his tongue was vibrating as I came, crying out loud until I flopped back down on the sofa.

He moved his mouth away and turned the egg off

before climbing up to join me. As I rested my head in his lap I congratulated myself on a good plan well executed. Adam, it was fair to say, was similarly pleased, which made me feel happy, and not unlike a goddess for a bit. Everyone wins.

Of course not all of my plans worked out quite as I had planned.

I'm a big fan of buying sex toys online. There are a couple of things I've bought in person, but mostly I'm internet all the way. No embarrassment (which is obviously a major thing with me – sadly even a trip to an Ann Summers shop can see me blushing), a great selection of items, lots of bargains and sales to be had and, usually, a good number of reviews that tell you how normal folk have found the objects you're considering buying. Invaluable stuff.

I have, however, on occasion not read the small print as well as perhaps I could have.

Adam and I had discussed anal play a lot. It was something he had a lot more experience of than me, and initially I was quite wary as my early experiences had been a mix of incredibly hot and quite painful. I decided I would order a plug for us to use together, something we could have fun with and that would act as a signal to Adam that I trusted him to do a little more arse-related stuff than we'd done previously.

As ever a victim of the allure of additional features and (non-literal) bells and whistles, I found one that could be inflated using a little bulb and that would vibrate as well. It was reasonably priced, a bargain even, and the fact it

73

could be made bigger seemed especially useful as I was getting used to having my bum played with.

When it arrived there was one problem.

I don't know whose arse it was supposed to fit into, but it wasn't going into mine, even before being expanded.

It was a bit ridiculous but made me laugh a lot. In an email to Adam I told him my mistake and explained how I was pondering sending it back for a refund (unused I hasten to add). Adam's email in response made me gulp a little bit.

Keep it. It might not be a total loss. x

Huh.

That Friday he came over and, as often happened, after an early dinner we spent the rest of the evening in bed.

At one point he asked to see the plug and I laughed as I fetched it. He said it was definitely too big to go in my arse, but that didn't mean it wouldn't fit elsewhere. I hid my nerves as best I could, but he just put it on the bedside table after inspecting it and we went back to debating who wrote the best Batman comics (Tim Sale, obviously, although he said Miller).

Gradually we became more amorous and half an hour later I had him in my mouth, slowly moving up and down, savouring the feeling as I knelt on the bed, his hand on my inner thigh.

I shivered as he ran his hand along my slit and then pushed a finger inside me. I moaned around his cock.

He withdrew and in a few moments I felt something else between my legs. He was pushing the plug into my cunt, presumably to show me that it wasn't a wasted purchase after all.

It was, somewhat disconcertingly, similar in shape to a cone, getting wider as he pushed it in. I groaned as he pushed the widest part inside me, feeling myself close around it. Just the thin shaft and base protruded. There were two cables attached – one to the controller for the vibration and one to the bulb that inflated it.

He immediately turned the vibration on to maximum, making me cry out at the sudden intensity. Then he squeezed the bulb. I felt the plug widen inside me. It was an odd sensation, not unpleasant, but it made me feel full.

But he wasn't done. He kept squeezing it, counting out loud the number of times he squeezed the bulb as he slowly inflated the toy inside me. He kept a hand on the base to prevent it from falling out and the pressure he put on it made it even more intense.

When he got to eight I was shaking. I kept my mouth on his cock but I had given up any hope of being able to pleasure him. I just knew he would want me to not let him slip out.

'Look at you, two of your holes filled at once. Do you like being nice and full?'

I really did. The intensity of the plug was on the very edge of being painful, but paired with sucking him (which remained one of my favourite things to do sexually) it was bringing me close to orgasm. That said, the sing-song nature of his voice irked me a little, so I ignored him.

He spanked my arse, hard enough that I was pretty sure he'd have left a hand print, and asked me again.

Grudgingly I nodded, unwilling to look at him, knowing that he'd be able to see how much I was enjoying it by how wet the bloody plug was.

'Do you think you'd enjoy it even more if all your holes were being used?'

I stiffened. Nervous. Unsure. We'd talked about triple penetration and I was very curious about it, although still half convinced most normal women wouldn't be able to cope with it, whatever the porn films said.

He didn't demand an answer from me this time, but I felt his finger moving around the toy, collecting as much of my juices as he could. He then began to circle my arse with his finger, making it wet. I couldn't help it, I went tense.

He stroked my arse, softly, giving me an odd kind of reassurance.

'It's OK, Sophie. I'm not going to hurt you, but if we're going to do this you need to relax or it might be uncomfortable.'

His finger returned to my opening, but stayed there.

'Push backwards for me sweetheart.'

I growled slightly around his cock and he laughed.

'I'm sorry, I promise I'm not doing it to be humiliating, it just means you can take this at your own pace.'

He might not have meant for it to be humiliating, but it still felt that way as I began to shift myself. I must have been incredibly wet, though, as my juices acted as a good lubricant as I moved backwards, my arse opening for his finger. It felt incredibly tight, undoubtedly because of the fullness in my cunt, but I was able to push back easily, allowing him to slide in.

As soon as his finger was inside me it was as though the vibrations of the toy were moving through it too. The feelings were incredibly intense. Any movement, however small, meant waves of pleasure pulsed through me, with even the movement of my body as I breathed in and out feeling powerful.

Adam started to thrust his hips upwards into my mouth. It reminded me that he was there and I began to lick him again, trying to focus on him as much as possible. It was pretty difficult with everything else going on. He pushed to the back of my throat and I gagged a little before taking him as far down as I could.

At that point he began to move his finger in and out, slowly at first but quickly getting faster and harder. I was moaning around his cock as he told me what a dirty girl I was for getting off on having all her holes used at once. I would have blushed if I wasn't already bright red.

He fucked my mouth, continuing his filthy monologue. Then he stopped mid-sentence and let out a cry. I felt him flood my mouth. As the first stream hit my tongue I too went over the edge, clamping my mouth round him as I bucked against his hand and the toy, my cries only muffled by his cock. I collapsed onto the bed. He withdrew his finger and quickly deflated the plug and turned it off, pulling it out of me.

It's ironic really because, while it didn't work very well as a plug for me, it became a toy that Adam particularly enjoyed using. My relationship with it veered between love and hate (depending on how far he expanded it) but, either way, when it came out of the toy drawer I knew life wouldn't be dull.

That said, it's not as if there was much chance for my life to be dull. A change in my job role made for slightly more regular hours, but while weekend shifts in the newsroom were a thankful rarity, later nights became more frequent. Paired with trips to see my parents every week or two, and keeping up with friends, life was always busy. My life was full before Adam arrived, but I was soon realising that I wanted to make room to fit him in it. I could see him enjoying the banter at my friends' birthday parties – complete with the drunken arguments about the hundred best albums ever recorded. I could see my parents liking him. Increasingly I realised my first instinct when I read or saw something interesting was to tell him.

It was odd.

It was lovely.

It made me nervous.

Post James I had decided I was not in the place for a relationship. But I felt myself wavering a little. Not for any relationship, and certainly not a relationship with James. But Adam. Straightforward, funny, clever, filthy Adam. That was very much a different thing.

I tried to tamp down the feelings as much as possible – not least because I felt somewhat guilty. We'd started this as a no-strings thing and while it hadn't been a conscious choice I was aware that the change in my feelings could make things awkward if he didn't feel the same. And, somewhat ironically, the one thing we weren't talking about at this juncture was our relationship – the sex, yes, previous relationships, yes, even what we wanted long term. Just not this. So, in true ostrich fashion, I just kept things as simple and straightforward as I could by, erm, not saying a word. I could mask the feelings, right?

According to Thomas I absolutely couldn't.

Adam and I had met him and Charlotte for dinner one

weeknight. It was a fun evening – lots of drinks, good banter, some nice food. Tom and Charlotte were both on good form, and by the time I'd said goodbye to the three of them to head home (Adam had an early start, making for a rare night where we didn't meet and then end up going home together) I had a stitch from laughing so hard.

When my phone pinged as I got to my car I assumed it would be Adam, saying goodnight (yes, we tended to do that too, but that's not a sign of anything and, I promise, isn't as sickening as it sounds). It wasn't.

Thomas says: You kept that quiet! I didn't realise things were that serious. Really pleased for you both though. About time.

I felt my face scrunch up in a mixture of confusion and scorn that, when she saw it, my mum always warned me would cause early wrinkles. What was he talking about? How did he know they were serious? *Were* they serious? According to whom? Had Adam said something to him?

Bearing in mind my ability to disappear off into an imaginative flight of fantasy with very little effort, I thought the best thing was to seek immediate clarification.

Sophie says: What do you mean, serious? Did Adam say something?

Hmmm. In hindsight that might have sounded a smidgen too keen, but curious minds need to know. Thankfully, Thomas didn't keep me in suspense too long.

Thomas says: Adam wouldn't say anything to me, and as far as I know, Charlotte hasn't asked him. I could ask her to if you want though.

Yikes. I replied as fast as my fingers would type.

Sophie says: No, no need to do that! So what did you mean then?

The reply pinged back almost immediately.

Thomas says: You're both clearly very happy. Charlotte says she's never seen Adam so obviously keen on a woman. And obviously I know you pretty well, and I'd hazard the same.

I couldn't help smiling. I know it's lame, looking to optimistic friends for relationship validation, but, hell, I'd take what I could get. I wasn't admitting that to him, though.

Sophie says: Yeah, yeah. You just want everyone as loved up as you two are.

There was no immediate reply – and one wasn't really needed – so finally I put my phone aside, buckled my seat belt and began the drive home. By the time I got back I had two messages waiting for me.

Thomas says: I wish we were loved up. Things aren't always what they seem.

I replied, asking him if he was OK, reminding him that if he ever wanted to chat I was here – let's face it, after everything we'd been through I knew him better than most, knew all about his kinky side, and wouldn't judge him for anything. He didn't respond.

As for the other message, as I tapped out a brief reply I sincerely hoped that WAS what it seemed.

Adam says: Miss you sweetheart. Really wish I could have stayed over tonight. Let me know you get back safely please. X

It was lame for me to feel a bit warm and fuzzy every time he called me 'sweetheart', right? I thought so.

Chapter Five

As mini-break-obsessed Bridget Jones knew, the first weekend away is a cornerstone of any new relationship. As far as I recall, though, hers didn't involve a St Andrew's Cross and mirrored ceilings.

Adam and I had been spending a lot of time together. There were still ridiculously early starts, where I packed him off with biscuits and a travel mug of coffee for a ninety-minute drive across the city to get to work. Paired with late nights interrupted with chat and lots of filthy sex, this meant we were in a constant state of smiling exhaustion.

My tiny flat was our bolthole. As we were both fundamentally antisocial, and were still in the heady days of wanting to jump each other at a second's notice, it made sense for him to come to mine rather than us going to his, with his (undoubtedly very nice) flatmate. But the flat, which was a fine size for one, suddenly felt constraining. I don't mean that I didn't enjoy sharing my space with Adam – if anything I was surprised how easily I took to having someone around so much after years of living alone. It was just, well, there weren't a huge amount of options for places to have sex other than the obvious bed and sofa, and the living room was, literally, not big enough to swing a cat-o-nine-tails. Although actually that might have been for the best – those things sting.

We were lying in bed one night when Adam suggested a

weekend away. As someone who, despite a lot of travelling with work, still remains tragically excited at the prospect of staying in hotels (oh, the free toiletries, breakfast in the restaurant, getting the paper delivered to your room, the minibar with overpriced yet tempting peanuts!), I agreed before he'd even fully explained what he was thinking of. And then when he did my brain was a little blown.

I think it's fair to say I'm not an especially innocent person, but even so I had never heard of the concept of a kink cottage. I knew you could hire out professional dungeons by the hour if you wanted, but the conveyor-belt nature of that (and my slight squeamishness about hygiene) meant it didn't really appeal to me, even to assuage my long-held curiosity and longer-held fantasies.

I was intrigued by the idea of playing in a dungeon, definitely, but frankly if I owned a house with lots of space the first thing I'd be doing with the big spare room in the basement would be building the best home cinema my budget would allow, rather than building a red room of pain. But apparently that's not a problem. You can rent whole kink-friendly holiday homes. I was fascinated. And also intrigued. We chose a weekend and Adam booked it. The details were scant, I think in part because he knew I would drive him crazy with questions about what we were going to do if I knew too much about the facilities beforehand, but he told me it was completely private, with lots of opportunities for rude fun and even a secluded garden in case we wanted to play outside. As a woman whose entire journey between work and home is covered by CCTV this intrigued me a lot, at least until the weekend arrived.

It was snowing. And not the 'throwing snowballs and drinking hot chocolate and having fun' snow, so much as the 'slushy, icy, miserable, you could break your neck walking to work and not be found until spring' snow. We had a debate about whether or not to go at all, but decided, having looked at the traffic information, that it was worth trying the two-hour drive to get there, not least because the cottage was likely to be warmer than my flat in winter, and Adam's booking for the weekend was non-refundable.

The drive up was one of nervous anticipation. We didn't talk much because Adam was concentrating on the road. While conditions weren't too treacherous, bad weather does make people drive like idiots and with the unknown roads he was even more vigilant than usual. The silence meant my mind wandered, and I began thinking about what I was letting myself in for, how things would go, whether it would be a long, intense experience or a series of short, sexy moments.

We found the cottage, tucked away at the end of a quiet residential road (I wonder if the neighbours suspected anything), as secluded as promised. We parked the car, picked up the key (hidden in a little pot by the door – ah, the joys of being out of the city) and unloaded our bags. I had a pretty hefty overnight bag, but barring clean clothes for the journey home, a washbag and phone charger it contained nothing but a series of outfits and underwear I had no intention of wearing outside the confines of our home for the next forty-eight hours. I dragged it inside and we wandered around the building, exploring.

Every room we walked through seemed to have some kind of kinky purpose to it, as I suppose you would expect. The living room had a St Andrew's Cross on the wall. I walked up to it the way you would an exhibit at an art gallery, looking at it with fascination, trying to imagine what it would feel like to be tied to it, seeing how sturdy it was. Adam was watching my reactions closely, perhaps too closely for my taste. He took my hand in his and pulled me towards the stairs.

'Maybe later.'

I felt my cheeks heat and he smiled; it made me smile back, secure in the knowledge that I could have fun here with him, that no matter how hardcore the setting, he wasn't going to metamorphose into some kind of über-dom who pushed me further than I could cope.

It was probably just as well I'd had that thought before I got to the top of the stairs, as the view from the landing made my throat go dry. Three closed doors led to more rooms, but my eyes were drawn to the cage, sitting neatly at the top of the stairs, the door open invitingly, a cushion and small blanket resting on the top of it.

Adam pushed open the first door, and I forced my feet to move, to follow him. A bathroom, with a bath big enough for two (OK, probably more than two, but certainly enough for us). The second door opened onto a huge bedroom dominated by a four-poster bed in dark wood complete with, I couldn't help but notice, metal rings attached at intervals along its main beams for bondage purposes. We put the bags on the floor and I trailed out behind Adam as he opened the door to the third room. I got a brief glimpse of a lot of equipment that looked not unlike a home gym, before the door was closed firmly again.

'Later,' he said again, his soft kiss on my nose conflicting with the familiar hungry look in his eyes. 'Let's get the rest of the bags first.'

We shuffled back downstairs, discovering the kitchen as we headed back to our starting point. The kitchen was the only room without any equipment or toys in it, and the thing that struck me most was how well equipped it was. Stainless-steel oven, hob and extractor fan, surfaces with plenty of space for cooking, a coffee machine, juice extractor. I peered into the oven. The whole place was pristine, which assuaged my concern about hygiene, but the kitchen was even cleaner than any of the other rooms. I suppose that made sense – who's spending a weekend in a kink cottage and making a roast instead? – but it seemed like a bit of a waste. Then I turned round and saw Adam's face, and all thoughts of cooking flitted from my head.

I was nervous and excited, watching him warily as he stood in front of me. Waiting. He'd brought two bags with him. He'd left the one containing his change of clothes upstairs. The other one, the soft black leather one I had grown to know well, the one that contained all his toys, was now clasped in his hands.

He was staring at me. Without breaking my gaze he unzipped his fly and pulled his cock out, beckoning me over in invitation. I smiled at him and took a step towards him, brought up short as he growled:

'No. Crawl.'

Suddenly the silence was really loud. I could feel my heart begin to beat faster. I gave him a dark look, but got on my hands and knees and crawled across the tiled kitchen floor, feeling faintly ridiculous in my jeans and jumper. When I reached him, I had a moment of doubt.

His cock was right there, but I didn't dare risk the presumption of taking him in my mouth. I looked up at him.

He laughed, and patted the side of my head. 'Good girl. You can suck me.'

I felt myself flush red, embarrassed that he'd taken it as a silent request for permission, even while I realised, with some surprise, that it really had been.

I took him gently in my mouth, sucking him softly, and he moaned, leaning against the counter. His sighs of pleasure as I began to use my tongue helped me recover my equilibrium a little. A sense of my own power returned as I watched him lose himself for a moment, his eyes fluttering shut as he enjoyed the feeling of my mouth on him.

It didn't last, though. He opened his eyes and, without looking down at me, he turned his body away from the counter top. I shifted with him, but he kept moving backwards, slowly walking across the room to the doorway and out of the kitchen.

He hadn't told me to keep him in my mouth, but the hint I took from his lack of speed paired with, frankly, the fact I didn't want to let him go, meant I crawled with him, even though it made me feel ungainly and a bit awkward. He led me through to the living room, then to the foot of the stairs. For a moment I thought he was going to walk up them backwards, and I was mentally pondering whether someone as naturally clumsy as me should in fact risk crawling up a flight of stairs while giving someone a blow job (what if I slipped? Potential mood killer at best and trip to accident and emergency at worst) when he reached down and grabbed me by a handful of my hair. He pulled me off his cock and up to my feet. I couldn't restrain a slight yelp.

He turned away to walk upstairs, tugging on my hair to make me follow. My scalp stung as I hurried after him into the kink room. I could barely take in my surroundings and all the items around me as he dragged me over towards the window and a pillory.

The first thing to say about the pillory is that a lot of people call them stocks. Technically – she says, sounding like a complete nerd – that's incorrect. Used as a form of punishment, criminals and ne'er-do-wells were held in stocks (which locked their feet in place) or pillories (their head and wrists) for public shaming. Rotten food was often thrown at them, and villagers would congregate to ridicule them – a kind of bonding experience and afternoon's entertainment all rolled into one for everyone except the poor bugger locked in place and the centre of attention. I've been fascinated with them since the first time I learned of their existence, in mediaeval history lessons in primary school. By the time I was studying history at A-level, I would lie in bed at night thinking of elaborate sexual fantasies whereby I'd be locked in a pillory, humiliated and fucked by any number of people who felt the urge to do so.

The pillory was one of my longest held sexual fantasies. I'd mentioned it to Adam months before, my voice halting and quiet in the darkness, embarrassed at not just the filth but also by how specific it was. But it was a kink I never anticipated getting to experience. I'd seen them in the odd museum over the years, but they tend to be old and rare; curators don't usually offer to let eager-eyed girls try them out, and frankly even if they did it's not as if you can indulge in any shenanigans in the middle of a museum or even at a historical re-enactments society shindig.

This one looked well-made of sturdy red wood. I found it oddly beautiful, and ran a finger along the smoothly varnished side, smiling to myself. Adam lifted the top off, exposing three curved grooves, a big one to rest my neck on and another two, one for each wrist. He grabbed me by the hair again, manoeuvring my neck into position. I hesitated for a moment, before putting my hands into the smaller grooves myself, allowing him to snap the top half back down, locking me into place.

My first feeling was a wave of panic, my second a surge of lust. Adam slotted in the piece of wood that held the two pieces together, and I was trapped. Properly trapped, against the unyielding cherry wood. It was difficult to move my head because of the weight on my neck, so my field of vision only reached to my feet and a small radius around them. I was bent at the waist, and the position was not only uncomfortable but made me feel incredibly vulnerable. My arse was sticking out and I could feel his eyes on me, his stare strong enough to make me feel naked. I was bloody grateful that I wasn't. Yet.

He moved round and stood in front of me, his cock so close to my face that I was breathing on it. Suddenly I understood why this pillory was lower than others I'd seen. It certainly made any twinge in my back at the uncomfortable position suddenly seem worthwhile.

He dropped his leather bag on the floor directly in my sightline, opened it up and began to rummage through it, although he did it in a way that meant – frustratingly – I didn't get too much of a glimpse of what was in there other than rope. And I figured that wasn't getting used here.

Finally he pulled out a small silver cylinder. A bullet

vibrator, maybe, was my first thought, but then he removed the top. Lipstick. I don't wear much make-up at all and am perfectly happy with lip balm for all but the biggest occasions, when I might wear a bit of gloss. I'm not a lipstick person, so this surprised me a little.

He twisted the base, revealing a bright-red hue. Really red. I looked at him suspiciously, and then he crouched down in front of me, brushing a few stray hairs out of my face and kissing me softly on the forehead. His touch was tender, soothing. All of which made what he did next even more jarring.

He took the lipstick and wrote something across my forehead. I was starting to tremble, my thoughts a maelstrom of embarrassment. It was a fair bet he'd written something horrible; I undoubtedly looked ridiculous. I also had a not-inconsiderable amount of fear that he'd bought one of those super-long-lasting lipsticks that would leave me with something degrading written on my forehead for ages. In my mounting hysteria I wondered whether I'd have to cut myself a fringe before I went to work on Monday.

'Do you know what it says?'

I shook my head, as much in an attempt to shake my hair in front of my face so he couldn't see the humiliation written there as to say no to his question.

'It says "whore".'

He knelt again, lifting my head up by pushing a finger under my chin, and brushed my hair away. But the atmosphere of the room had changed. I no longer felt tenderness, just the sting of humiliation. It burned, brighter and brighter, as he began coating my lips with the bold lipstick, his fingers pinching at my chin as he circled my mouth over and over again. By the time he was done I must have looked like a clown. My lips felt sticky and swollen, not my own.

He walked behind me, but the relief I felt at him disappearing from my field of vision lasted barely a second before his hands snaked around my waist, unfastening my trousers and pulling them to my knees, along with my knickers. I shuffled my legs to try and step out of them but Adam slapped my arse in warning. The feeling of being half undressed, displayed in that way, made me feel more vulnerable than if I had been totally naked, but then I felt a tickle as he began writing on my arse, and my legs began to shake.

'In case you're wondering, it says "slut".' I felt a surge of fury. He moved back to face me, and without any warning grabbed my hair and pulled my mouth onto his cock, pushing himself in and pulling my hair until he was so deep I began to choke, struggling to breathe. I felt my fingers moving in desperation, immobilised in their little wooden holes, trying to move, to pull him back.

Just as quickly he pulled back, leaving me staring at his cock, which was smeared with lipstick and glistening with my saliva. He moved closer, and I opened my mouth, expecting him to push himself inside me again, but instead he showed me the line where the lipstick stopped, around three-quarters of the way down his shaft.

'You need to try harder,' he said as he pushed himself back in.

I understood the game, and tried to open my mouth wider to allow him deeper, but within a few seconds panic rose and I was choking again, my eyes beginning to water. He pulled back, leaving a line of saliva stretching from my mouth to the tip of his cock. I closed my eyes as I saw it, whimpering slightly in embarrassment. He looked down to see the cause of my distress, and casually moved forward again, wiping himself on my cheek before checking again for where the mark was. I kept my eyes resolutely closed, not wanting to give him the satisfaction of seeing that I was finding the humiliation so intense my eyes had turned from watering to tearful. Much to my relief, he let it go. For now.

'That's better, but you're still not quite there. One last effort. Come on, sweetheart.'

His words spurred me on. I took a deep breath in the moment before he thrust back into my mouth. I fought my gag reflex, trying to quell the rising panic at being unable to breathe and somehow, despite the odd angle and my nerves, his cock slid down my throat. His groan was loud and made me feel a surge of pride. I held myself completely still, struggling to breathe through my nose which was pressed into his groin. I managed it for a few seconds, but eventually I began to choke again and he pulled out, nonchalantly wiping the combined pre-cum and saliva around my face. As he moved closer to my cheek I saw the lipstick all the way down his shaft. My competitive spirit felt like this was a win, which is ridiculous when you remember the position I was in, but I guess we have to take our victories where we can get them. I tried to gloss over what a mess my face must have looked by then.

He began to push himself into my mouth again, hard.

He grabbed handfuls of my hair, pulling my head up as far as the pillory would let me, keeping me in place so he could thrust in and out in a mockery of the rhythm he would use to fuck me. At times I gagged and choked, but more often he slipped down into my throat, until he pulled out abruptly and began stroking himself really fast, right in front of my face. I knew him well enough now to know when an orgasm was impending, and to my frustration and annoyance he came, with a deep groan. I closed my eyes, but could do nothing to stop him coming in my face and hair.

When I opened my eyes he was tucking himself back in his trousers and looking down at me. He reached down and opened the pillory. I slowly stood up, stretching a little to ease the ache in my shoulders. I was confused. Was that the end for now? But then he grabbed me by the hair, being careful not to get cum on his hand, and pulled me out of the room and into the hallway, allowing me to step out of my trousers and knickers – finally – as I walked, and removing my blouse and bra in a businesslike fashion at the same time. I felt some of his cum drip from my chin onto my breasts as I followed. He led me to the cage.

We stood looking at it for long moments. I have been intrigued by cages and cells for a long time, dating back to my earliest fascination with Maid Marian, held captive by Guy of Gisborne and the Sherriff of Nottingham in their ongoing battle to catch Robin Hood. But standing in front of one, knowing Adam was waiting for me to crawl into it, I felt nervous. Suddenly it felt like a leap over the precipice to clamber inside. To do so willingly. I looked up at him, watching him look at the cage, wondering what he was thinking. And then his gaze flickered to mine, and the moment for pause had passed.

He tugged on my hair, pulling me towards the cage, gesturing with his head. Slowly I got back onto all fours, pausing for a moment to figure out the best way to get in and be comfortable.

It wasn't a large cage. Four feet at its highest; its length and sides were slightly smaller. The bars were thick and made of unyielding-looking steel, wide enough to get a couple of fingers between them but nothing more.

He opened the door and threw the cushion onto the floor, pushing me with his foot towards the entrance. I shifted slightly, turning myself so that I went in backwards, still able to face him as I did so, trying to maintain my modesty by not giving him a face-on view of exactly how wet my treatment in the pillory had made me.

I shuffled in, settling onto the cushion on my hands and knees waiting to see what he would do next. The answer was 'not much'. He closed and locked the door from the outside and then walked back downstairs.

'Call me if you need anything.'

His words confused me a little. It was pretty obvious that what I needed, more than anything else, was a chance to come. Did he not mean that? Did he want me to ask for that? Or did he want me to stay quiet and wait? How long *would* I wait?

I stayed knelt up for a few minutes, certain he would return with something from his bag of tricks, or to do something else to me, to continue the game. Instead I heard him walk to the kitchen, the sound of the fridge opening and closing, and then the sound of the TV being switched on. He was clearly planning on leaving me here for a while. The thought made me furious – the idea he would use me and then basically lock me up until he was ready to do more fiendish things with me, as if I was a toy. But the more I thought about it, the wetter it made me, which left me confused as much as aroused. I curled into a ball on my side, keeping my eyes on the top of the stairs, but also enjoying the peace and the freedom of it. I know that sounds crazy, but there was something very relaxing and freeing about it. The hallway was warm, I had my cushion to keep me comfy. I found myself staring at the bars, reaching out to touch them.

After a while I closed my eyes, reliving what had happened, how being in the pillory had felt, blushing a little at how aroused it had made me, even with the embarrassment and anger. The adrenaline from the intensity of his treatment, the face fucking and the humiliation, began to dissipate and I began to feel sleepy in the warmth of the corridor. I drifted off, enjoying the fact I had nowhere else to be, nothing else to do. I was literally lying there waiting for him to come back so we could have more kinky sex. It's not something I'd want to be the focus of my world the entire time, but for this little while, there were definitely worse places to be.

He made me jump when he opened the door. I had no idea how long I'd been dozing, but I hadn't heard his return upstairs. He beckoned me out, offering me his arm to help me stand up, solicitously leading me down the stairs in case my legs were stiff from being bent for so long. I followed him nervously, feeling shy and self-conscious, knowing that I had his dried cum and the lipstick all over my face.

My heart began to pound as I saw the scene in front of me. The St Andrew's Cross had been moved to the centre of the room and next to it was his crop. Seeing it surprised me – when he'd arrived with two bags I'd assumed he'd brought something else because I knew the crop wouldn't fit in either of them. He must have hidden it somewhere in the car and retrieved it later. Shit.

I stole a glance at his face. There was no humour in his eyes, just a stern, assessing gaze, as if he was measuring me for something. Fleetingly I wondered, worried, if I was going to be found wanting. It had been a long time since I'd been really hurt. Adam was much more about psychology and humiliation rather than pain. He had only used the crop on me briefly once before and spanked me a few times, although he joked that his hand got tired before I got too uncomfortable, my reputation as a pain slut apparently still intact.

He turned me around to face the cross, using cuffs to fasten me in position at the wrists and ankles, leaving my arms and legs spread open.

I was trying to prepare myself for the pain, aware that if he wanted to do more than a peremptory few swats this was going to hurt. He was taking his time, though. He ran the end of his crop up and down my back and between my legs, chuckling as I flinched. He left the crop there for a few terrifying seconds, my thigh muscles trembling as I fought to close my legs. I couldn't, of course. Trust me: at that moment if I could have I would have. He pulled the crop back.

'Your juices are sticking to it. Well, I guess that answers the question about how much you enjoyed the pillory and the cage.'

I flushed. He was right. In another context (probably later, with tea and a biscuit) I'd be able to admit what we both already knew, that being treated this way, hurt, humiliated, locked up, was making me incredibly turned on. We'd even be able to talk rationally about what felt most hot, most challenging. But not now. Right now, listing to his stern and imperious voice, I was embarrassed, shy and oddly furious at how gleeful he was at how wet this was making me. Even though I *was* wet, and we were both enjoying it, I felt the need to lash out a little.

Turns out it wasn't me that was going to be doing the lashing.

'You're going to count down from fifty.'

What? Shit. The terror started then. The crop produced an intense pain – he had only used it on me once before, and I'd not taken anything like fifty strikes from it. I wasn't sure how I could. Maybe it was just as well the cuffs were holding my ankles in place. Then I felt a few seconds of wild optimism. Maybe he meant he wanted me to count down to fifty before he started cropping me, maybe he was messing with my mind, building the anticip–

The first strike hit my arse. Fuck. OK. The adrenaline started again. Fine. Let's do this.

'Fifty.'

He hit me again. And again. And again. And again.

The first ten stung a bit, but he was clearly holding back. I began to think I could maybe endure this, if this was the level he was going to keep it at.

97

Of course he wasn't. Even I think I'm an idiot in hind-sight, but clearly I'm an optimist at heart.

The next ten actively hurt.

The five after that made me cry out.

The next five made me cry, tears streaming down my face in a way which, I realised later, just made my face look more of a mess, although at the time I didn't have the capacity to be aware of it in my struggle to cope with the strikes.

The final twenty were a huge challenge. He hit harder and harder, the sound of the crop whistling through the air in a way that filled me with fear. My arse and thighs were on fire, and when I didn't say the numbers fast enough between soft sobs he would make me count them again. And again if need be. By the time he finally finished I had probably been hit more like seventy times.

When I finally reached number one, my body shook with relief. Adam quickly freed me from the cross and eased me down onto the floor, so that I avoided sitting on my burning bum. He sat with me, my head in his lap as he stroked my hair, letting the reaction move through me like a tropical rainstorm both in its intensity and the speed with which it passed.

He whispered into my ear as I got my breath back, his voice calming. He told me how wonderful I was, how pleased he was with me for enduring the crop so beauti-fully for him. How lovely the marks on my arse looked. How proud he was of me. How impressed at my bravery. His words warmed me, soothed me, as did the endorphins running through my body and my relief at having not just endured for him but done well. My breathing slowed. I calmed down. And suddenly I was just a very dishevelled-looking woman with a pleasingly warm arse and an incredibly wet cunt.

He smiled down at me.

'Would you like to come now?'

I nodded quickly, feeling myself flush a little at my eagerness. 'Yes please.'

Gently he helped me up. He took my hand and led me back upstairs to the bedroom.

He pulled me down onto the bed, kissing me passionately. Our tongues tangled, our hands were everywhere. The dynamic had changed to something more playful. This was Adam as I knew him most often: still with moments of danger, but mostly lovely, sensual. Loving. He pulled away for a moment to smile down at me and I saw the redness around his lips and remembered the lipstick on my face. The room had large mirrors on each wall and the ceiling, and I snuck a glance in the nearest one, groaning quietly as I saw the red smudges, dried cum and the faint imprint of 'whore' reflected backwards across my forehead.

I'd always thought mirrors were a bit too Playboy Mansion for my taste, but in this room they gave almost a 360° view of everything, which I liked, although it made it difficult to ignore the things that I found challenging (my possibly stained forehead), at least until I began to watch Adam strip in the mirror. He was finally taking off his clothes and giving me an unimpeded view of his hard cock, and then his arse as he leaned down to retrieve a condom from his bag.

When he was finally naked and ready he moved me onto my hands and knees and slid inside me from behind.

I let out a long groan of pleasure as he began to roughly fuck me – after so much teasing and so many intense experiences in such a relatively short length of time I was more than ready for this.

He grabbed a handful of my hair and began to use it as leverage, pulling me back onto him as fast as he pushed into me. His thrusts gave me a paradoxical mix of pain and pleasure. My arse and thighs were still stinging from the crop, and feeling him bash against them with every movement brought new waves of searing heat from the welts, but that was paired with the pleasure of feeling him inside me. It felt amazing.

His hands pulled my head up and made me arch my back, which meant I could see my own face in the mirror again. I flushed at the wanton, dishevelled mess he had rendered me, shocked at the lust in my eyes and the smile of joy on my face. My expression brought me up short for a moment; it was a rare visual insight into how I looked during my own submission. I was surprised by how happy I looked – no grumpy face here – and also how I seemed younger and more carefree somehow.

I was suddenly dragged back into the moment by the movement behind me. My eyes flickered to Adam, my tormentor, my partner in crime, the man who had very quietly done everything he could to fulfil lots of my longest-held fantasies. I watched him as we fucked, enjoying the look of concentration and lust in his eyes as I felt him slide in and out of me.

After a while he pulled out, manoeuvring me across the bed onto my back before beginning to fuck me again. His weight pressing my arse into the sheets, the welts rubbing across the soft cotton as we moved, made for even more pain, but by that point I didn't care – I was concentrating on looking over his shoulder in the mirror, watching him push in and out of me, seeing the point where we were joined so intimately.

The combination of the pain, the pleasure and the voyeuristic feeling of watching ourselves in mirrors meant I was so close to orgasm that my thighs were shaking with the effort of fending it off. In my submissive headspace it felt, more than ever, like something I should ask for. I did so, my voice sounding desperate even to my own ears, my relief when he said 'of course' almost a tangible thing.

I came. Hard. Once I had stopped trembling he climbed off me and lay on his back next to me on the bed while I recovered, his hand stroking my arm, creating a moment of connection that helped finally ground me, bringing me back down to earth.

When my breathing finally stilled I turned to crawl into his arms, but as I did so I saw his cock, hard and covered in my juices.

I know he'd taken his pleasure and left me unsatisfied in the cage, but I clearly was a nicer person than him and didn't want to see him denied. OK, mostly his cock looked tempting and I really wanted him to come in my mouth – I'm not that selfless. I looked over, to check he had no more plans for now and wasn't going to stop me. He smiled, and put his hands behind his head, a silent indication that he wasn't going to interrupt me now. It was my turn to play.

While I knew that he had enjoyed the things we'd done that afternoon, the knowledge that he'd taken so much effort doing them for me, knowing how much I wanted to try them, made my heart feel full. I wanted to do something for him, something that I knew he'd like.

I crawled down the bed and took him in my mouth, and where I'd tried to hide my arousal and indignity when getting into the cage, I now revelled in it, showed it to him. I positioned myself so that he could see my red and bruised arse while I sucked him, so he could see not just how wet I already was, but how doing this for him made me even wetter.

For now the flurry of violence and roughness had passed. He didn't fuck my face or hold my head down. He lay, watching me intently – I have a sneaking suspicion his eyes might have flickered to the mirror in front – as I sucked him. I gave myself to him eagerly, taking him as far into my mouth as I could, managing to slide him into my throat by myself, giving rather than letting him take it. Every time I did so I smiled to myself as I heard his groan. I loved the fact that I felt him throb in my mouth. Finally, when he came, I made sure to swallow every last drop. Then, and only then, I crawled back into his arms, pressed a kiss to his chest and began to doze.

When I stirred again, woken by Adam disentangling himself and slipping outside, the room was almost dark. I lay enjoying the warmth of the duvet for a little longer before getting up to explore. I found him in the bathroom, his hair damp from the shower, running me a bath. He helped me into it, kissing me softly and smiling as I sighed in pleasure at the warm water soothing my aches and pain.

He went off to get dressed, returning to bring me the

washbag containing my shampoo and shower gel, and the paperback I was currently carrying around in my handbag for rare moments of peace. He knelt by the bath and kissed me again, before telling me he was going to sort out dinner and I should have a leisurely bath before getting dressed and coming back downstairs to eat.

I was exhausted, blissed out, enjoying the simple pleasure of my bath after the intensity of everything that had gone before. I nodded and smiled as he leaned down to whisper in my ear:

'You should probably make sure you scrub that writing off your face and arse.'

He left the room whistling. I would have thrown my paperback after him, but what would I have had to read then?

After a good few chapters and rinsing myself clean of bubbles with the kind of decadently lengthy shower you'd never have at home lest you used all the hot water, I slipped on trousers and a jumper and went downstairs.

'Your timing is perfect,' he called from the kitchen. 'Settle down on the sofa. I'll bring the food in.'

The fire was on, the curtains drawn, the TV flickering in the background. I sat on the black leather sofa (presumably easier to wipe clean, although I probably didn't want to think about that then) and watched as Adam padded back into the room carrying two plates. He placed them down with a flourish, and I laughed as I took in the sight of two paper wrappings of takeaway fish and chips, complete with mushy peas for me. He disappeared to return again, this time carrying cutlery, salt, and a bottle of champagne and two glasses. He fiddled with the TV remote and the copyright screen for a DVD flickered on the screen – I laughed to see he'd thought to pack *The Shield* box set we'd been slowly working through.

We ate our fish and chips from the paper, drank champagne and curled up together on the sofa chatting about random things. It was fun, lovely, simple, and after the intensity of everything that had happened earlier that day, just perfect. My final thought as I drifted off to sleep was of simple joy and gratefulness for Adam's rudeness and kindness.

We spent great chunks of the rest of the weekend fucking like rabbits. With snow on the ground it was most definitely too cold to play outside, much to my disappointment. But we had sex in the deep-filled bath (tougher than I imagined, and not just for the mopping up of spilled water afterwards) and in front of the fire (a bit of a seventies porn film vibe admittedly but lovely). We went back to the pillory where I had an intense orgasm while held in position, although we realised there were practical problems when you have a woman whose legs go wobbly when she's orgasming being held up purely by her neck and wrists – it was slightly less alluring when Adam was having to hold me up to stop me choking by accident. We played doctor and patient complete with a chair with stirrups and non-NHS regulation straps. He tied me to the bed – and kept me under it in a cage we discovered the second night, although he took pity on me and let me back under the covers with him to actually go to sleep. I loved sleeping in his arms, but wished we were staying longer so I could experience more. Experience everything.

We watched more episodes of *The Shield* when we needed a rest from rudeness. I was incredulous I had missed a show both so good and with so many episodes. I cooked a fry-up. Adam made fajitas with homemade salsa so good it made me swoon. We drank tea. Read the papers. These small moments of cohabitation felt easy, comfortable, wonderful. Worryingly, they also felt a little like the beginning of a real relationship, the one we had both said we weren't interested in having. My internal monologue was trying to warn me, but mostly I didn't care.

At one unguarded moment on Sunday morning, I put my foot in it. I'd made breakfast, and was carrying it in to the table while Adam made space in between piles of newspaper supplements.

'It's funny, this is the best stuff about being in a relationship, these lazy moments with the papers, being comfortable not doing much.'

He looked up at me from folding the sports supplement and I suddenly realised my faux pas. I headed back to the kitchen to grab the coffees, fumbling desperately to underplay what I'd just said.

'Not that we're *in* a relationship, obviously. We did agree this was going to be a casual thing.'

He put the papers down and took a mug from my hand, kissing me gently as he did so.

'You're right, we did say this was going to be a casual thing.'

Bum. I put my coffee down and fled for the tomato sauce to give myself a second to school my features before returning to the table.

As I did, he spoke. 'But this doesn't feel casual to me. Laid-back, yes. Fun, definitely. But I think it's gone past casual, don't you?'

I took a long look at him before I replied. I was pretty sure this wasn't a trick question, but there was still a moment's pause before I answered. 'Yes.'

He grinned at me. 'Shall we work on the basis that this is now a proper relationship then? That we're partners or boyfriend and girlfriend or whatever you want to call it?'

I nodded.

'OK. Well, now we've got that sorted, shall we eat breakfast?' he asked, presumably nonplussed at the lunatic woman grinning at him and clutching a bottle of ketchup.

I nodded again.

'Well, come on then. Eat your breakfast.'

I did. I needed to keep my strength up for the rest of the weekend, after all.

Chapter Six

So we were officially dating. I say 'officially' but it's not like we put out a memo, or that it changed anything much. We spent more weekends together, our busy family and social lives allowing, but otherwise we continued seeing each other, fucking each other senseless whenever we had the time and privacy to do so, emailing and texting messages about politics and TV, and having random chats about our lives during the day.

There was no drama or fuss, no worrying about whether Adam would call or not, or what he meant as opposed to what he said, because he was so straightforward that he encouraged similar honesty. We talked about anything and everything: family, work trouble (including a pretty difficult time where, like most of the journalism industry in the last few years, I found myself at risk of redundancy), how we wanted to live our lives. We also talked more frankly than I ever have before about sex. I know, be afraid! It's hardly as if I'm backwards about coming forwards with this stuff anyway.

It was liberating, though, to have a boyfriend (although calling him that still felt very juvenile, while 'partner' was just a bit hippyish) who not only was completely open-minded about my sexuality, but also revelled in it. He loved me talking about what turned me on, the things I thought about as I touched myself lying in bed at night.

I told him everything. The things that made me blush. The things that made me wet. The fantasies so dark that I'd probably never do them in real life, but that under cover of darkness we could whisper to each other, not only safe in the knowledge we wouldn't judge each other, but that we would actively find it hot. Having spent so much of my life wondering how you find a guy who would not freak out at what, to some, would seem like a dark sexuality (although I still maintain I'm pretty sedate on the whole smut scale, it's just not many of us talk about it so freely), it was wonderful to be able to enjoy that side of things with Adam, and then re-watch *Homeland* together on DVD, make pancakes in funny shapes or play Scrabble until the early hours.

We'd settled into a routine, and it was wonderful. And then one day, shortly before the Easter holiday, I got a phone call from my mum. She was crying. My mum never cries at real life. Adverts, or those terrible made-for-TV movies they show on Channel Five of an afternoon all about alcoholic parents or children succumbing to cancer, yes, but in real life she is one of the toughest and most capable women I know.

She'd had a fall while clearing the guttering of leaves and had broken her knee. They were taking her into emergency surgery, but she wasn't sure what was going to happen afterwards.

Normally, it would have been a no-brainer. My parents have been married almost forty years and are devoted to each other. But my dad had, that morning, got on a plane to Hong Kong for a week's business trip. It had taken months to organise. Normally my brother would be around to help out – not least because he lived nearer – but he was on a month's work placement in the US, working hard for a promotion. My mum, with a lifetime of never being a bother behind her, was distraught at the thought of asking either of them to change their plans.

I'm incredibly close to all of my immediate family. There was no question as to what I would do. Thankfully I had some time off already booked over the long weekend, and enough hours owed (and a kind enough news editor) that with a bit of re-jigging I suddenly had nine straight days free to head back to my parents' house. I nipped home to grab some clothes, toiletries and my laptop, stopping long enough to ring my dad and brother and let them know that Mum was fine and I was on my way to the hospital to be with her when she got out of surgery. I also called Adam to tell him our smutty plans for the weekend were on hold. Then I set off.

Of course the thing about operations is that there is a lot of waiting around. I burst into the hospital reception in a fluster, to find that my mum wasn't going to be out of surgery for at least another few hours. I sat in the waiting room, fielding calls of concern, feeling ever more tense, and finally, finally, someone came through to tell me she was out. I think I must have looked like I was having a bit of a breakdown, because they told me that once she had emerged from the anaesthetic and gone up to a ward for the night they'd let me in to see her, despite the fact we were past hospital visiting hours.

Seeing her was a blessed relief. Suddenly I was aware, in that way you only really are when something like this happens, that despite the fact I felt so immature that some days I couldn't decide what to have for dinner, both my parents and I were ageing and there might be a time when they weren't around any longer. I held her hand, and she smiled at me sleepily, looking pale and poorly but with enough of a twinkle in her eyes to ease my fears. I kissed her gently and then headed back to my parents' house for the night to do the ring round of family members and friends with the update on her condition (for once I wished my mum would join Facebook, just to make it easier). I packed her a bag for the morning and started Mum-proofing things so she could cope when she came home.

She came home sooner than I expected. Arguably too soon, although I can't complain about the quality of care she got while she was in hospital, just that they seemed keen to get her out of the bed and the next person in. Two days after her surgery I was helping her, oh so slowly, get to my car on her crutches, driving her home carefully, cursing every pothole that made the car move in a way that jarred her knee and made her wince. She was in a lot of pain, taking five kinds of drugs in four different batches through the day. Walking hurt, sitting hurt, she couldn't climb into or out of bed without help. She veered from being irritable at needing help to weepily grateful, because she knew she couldn't do it without me.

In the dark first days after her operation we were the centre of each other's worlds. I slept next to her, so I could help her get up and to the bathroom if she needed to in the night. I got up when she did, went to bed when she did (although I didn't sleep – sleep wasn't coming eas-ily), cooked all her meals, helped her with her pills, talked her through her mood swings, mopped up her tears, reassured her when she was worried something had gone wrong. It was all-encompassing and exhausting and I'm not mentioning it in order to brag. The one thing the week taught me was that even with someone I love I am not a natural nurse. I am too impatient and easily frustrated. Also, lack of sleep makes me crazy.

There was no time for fun or frivolity. Even my current affairs obsession slipped, and I found myself reading the paper at ten o'clock at night, if at all. I spoke to Adam briefly on the phone a couple of nights in, but caught myself tearfully telling him the difficulties of helping Mum get back and forth from the bathroom and keeping on top of her pill cycle in such depth that I thought it was best not to inflict it on him again, not least because he was going to work, having his weekends and generally going about his life as normal. Also, if I'm honest, it scared me how much just hearing his voice made things feel better. This wasn't something I should be relying on him to help me through. I should be able to do this on my own. Well, that was my logic at least.

My logic was bollocks.

As the days went by things got easier. My mum began to make progress. She was more sure on her feet. Getting up and downstairs on her crutches was speedier. As she began to heal, the pain became a little easier, meaning she was more her usual self. Her appetite picked up, so I felt less like a contestant on *Masterchef* who put in loads of work and then had their culinary creations cast aside after a couple of mouthfuls. And then my dad came home, and the look of joy and relief on my mum's face was obvious.

By the time I packed up my car and drove back to my flat ready for my return to work I was exhausted. The stress hadn't eased, and I still felt bad for my poor mum. And when I walked through the door and found nine-day-old washing-up in my sink and work clothes waiting to be washed, my heart sank. I pushed myself to get through it all and then went to bed at 1 a.m. before a 7 a.m. shift, cursing myself for being a disorganised idiot.

Things, of course, got easier. I've never before had a holiday where a return to work felt like a relief, but in this case it did. As I got back into the routine of work, the stress I had felt mostly cleared. But there was one weird thing that had happened somewhere along the way, and I couldn't figure out how or when or why, but it was starting to get me worried.

I'm pretty highly sexed. This book is a fairly good sign of that, even with the caveat that it's mostly about my sex life rather than all the other stuff I do (I could write a book about my love of drinking tea, doing Sudoku and watching reruns of *The Big Bang Theory* but I don't think it'd be of similarly broad appeal). Since I'd started seeing Adam we'd been managing to have sex pretty much twice a day when we were together, often even more than that. But even when I wasn't dating the only man I'd ever met who could keep up with me on that front, I had a routine. Every night I had an orgasm lying in bed before I went to sleep. You can keep your hot milk or your sheep counting or whatever it is you do, an orgasm is by far the most efficient way to get me to sleep of a night.

But I hadn't had an orgasm for a while. I counted it. Nine days. Initially it was because I was sleeping in the bed with my mum and, well, that would be rather disturbing. Even when she was recovered enough that I moved down the corridor to my old childhood bedroom it didn't happen. I fell into bed exhausted, slept fitfully, but even when I tried . . . nothing.

I put it down to stress and tension, and tried not to worry about it, but once I'd returned home and had a couple of days back at work, I tried all the tricks (hot baths, smutty books on the Kindle, flirty emails with Adam) and nothing was doing the job. It was all incredibly fun, but there was just no release. I had been touching myself like this nightly (barring shared bedrooms and other inappropriate/inconvenient circumstances) literally since I was old enough to discover what an orgasm was, but suddenly it was like my body was a stranger. Nothing worked.

Nine days became ten. Eleven. By twelve days I was beginning to panic. This wasn't like me. Not only was I irritable at work and sleep deprived because it took me ages to drift off at night, but I was genuinely worried. While I knew Adam well enough to know our relationship wasn't all about sex, it formed a pretty decent foundation to it. What happens when you have a girlfriend who can't orgasm?

I was soon to find out.

I told him about it on the phone. He'd rung one day to see how I was doing. It was unusual, because normally we talked constantly via text, email or Messenger, saving our chat for in person during the weekends or weeknights we were together (although a crazy few weeks at work for him meant midweek visits hadn't happened either). I was so pleased to hear his voice, though also admittedly terrified – how DO you tell your boyfriend that you've gone from being a high-libido, kinky sex-obsessed erotica writer to someone who hasn't orgasmed for the best part of a fortnight? And is it even possible to do so without crying? In my case, no. It was the first time I'd cried in front of him and I felt like a melodramatic idiot. And he was lovely about it, which just made me more weepy.

He told me to stop trying, to try to stop worrying, and to come round for the weekend, starting the following night. His flatmate was going to be out until late on Sunday at a stag do, so we could have the place to ourselves. He would look after me for a bit, and I could just catch up on sleep, relax and try and regain my equilibrium.

Frankly I wasn't sure it was going to work, but short of finding a tumble dryer to sit on I was out of ideas.

I arrived at his house flustered and already, if I'm honest, a little grumpy. Work had been busy, and my day had been filled with minor annoyances. A great chunk of the afternoon had been spent discussing a complaint made by the subject of a story I'd written and which had caused a lot of reader feedback. I could prove that he had said what he'd said and I hadn't misquoted him, but the effort involved in digging out the Dictaphone tape, playing it to first my editor and then my managing editor, and then coming up with a response to the complaint meant that by the time I got out I was craving red wine. Preferably in my flat alone, not least because, having not seen Adam for almost three weeks by this point, I wanted to be sociable, friendly, fun and not an idiot the next time he saw me.

I'm not sure I was any of those but he did give me a big

glass of wine. Seeing him as he opened the door, I felt a surge of butterflies. It wasn't just the usual lust; it was also affection. I fell into him, squeezing him back as he hugged me tightly, leaning eagerly into his kiss hello, opening my mouth to urge his tongue deeper.

He gave me lots of attention and fuss. He made me toad-in-the-hole and mustard mash, the kind of comforting dinner that was perfect for a chilly Friday night, especially when combined with good company. He kept the conversation light, noticeably focusing on trying to make me laugh. He offered me chocolate mousse (it would have been rude to decline) and a glass of good port, and we settled in to watch a film on DVD, taking our glasses to the sofa. As the minutes ticked by I began to feel tired, resting my head on his chest. He put his arm round me and everything felt right. Lovely, actually.

When the film finished he took my hand and led me into the bedroom. I was feeling nervous, but not in the usual D/s-ish way. This was more a kind of performance anxiety I suppose. I was torn. This was Adam, lovely, sexy, wonderful Adam, who I hadn't seen for ages. I wanted to jump his bones, but at the same time I was desperately wondering if I could plead sleep or feign tiredness to avoid the potential awkwardness of what might happen next.

He wrapped his arms round me and began kissing me again. Soft, gentle brushes of his lips with mine to start with, developing into a passionate kiss, his tongue pushing inside my mouth, while his hands stroked my back.

He broke away to lift my top over my head, pulling me back to kiss me again, as if he didn't want to stop until he had to, or was worried about breaking the spell. I'd not kissed anyone as much as I had kissed Adam, and it was wonderful, romantic, gentle. Our mouths stayed glued together as he unfastened my bra. When his hands moved to my waist I mirrored his movements, and, still kissing, we unfastened each other's jeans.

He broke the kiss once more to pull my bra down my arms and lift his own T-shirt over his head. I couldn't stop myself grinning at him as I drank in the sight of him naked, and the last thing I saw before he moved back in to kiss me again was his own smile reflected back at me.

He walked me backwards until the back of my legs met the bed, then put gentle pressure on my shoulders to first sit and then lie me down. As I moved backwards he followed me, the tip of his cock brushing my thigh, making me shiver.

When his lips finally left mine he kissed my cheek, and then took my earlobe between his teeth, gently nibbling before moving lower. He kissed my neck and chest, reacquainting himself with my breasts, caressing them, softly licking and sucking on my nipples.

He continued down my stomach, making sure not to miss an inch of my skin. I spread my legs in lewd invitation, but he began kissing down my inner thigh instead. I moaned, in pleasure but also in frustration. I knew I was wet (which had to be a good start, right?) and I wanted him to taste me.

He kissed down to my knee and then shifted to the other leg, kissing back up. As he got close to where I was so desperate for him to be, I held my breath. I felt his warm breath on my wetness and it gave me goosebumps.

I was trembling with anticipation and eventually, finally, I felt his tongue on me. One long lick from my opening to my clit. I almost shouted with joy and relief.

He took his time, licking with the flat of his tongue over and over again before using the tip to move up and down my lips. Then he fucked me with his mouth. My eyes closed and my head went back as he pushed inside, his tongue entering me as deep as it could, his face pressed against me, coated in my juices.

He moved his tongue, his intimate kisses an echo of the passionate kisses that had left my mouth swollen just minutes before. It felt sensual, amazing, and I was shocked to feel how it had affected me. I was incredibly wet, audibly so. The idea might have made me blush earlier in the evening but I tried to push that away, to lie back and lose myself to the wonderful feelings he was evoking.

I don't know how long he licked me, just that it was a long time, but still didn't feel long enough. Eventually he moved his mouth and began licking my clit. He licked and sucked, getting harder and faster. I felt myself get closer and closer to orgasm, but as fast as the thought filled my mind the feeling dissipated. Suddenly non-rude thoughts entered my head. All the stressful things I'd been thinking about were there, my worries about whether this would work, the bone-weary tiredness. I knew I wouldn't come now, and I had no idea why that was or how to get past it. And I knew he'd be disappointed and I hated that too, because he'd been so lovely and done everything he could to make the night special and it wasn't enough. I wanted to cry.

I pulled back away from him, and for the first time ever

it wasn't playful or bratty, it was real. I just couldn't. Being somewhat busy and thus oblivious to my change in mindset Adam tried to follow me with his mouth. I had to push him away at the shoulder and tell him to stop. He looked up at me, confused.

'I'm sorry, I just don't think I can. It's not that I don't want to. God, I really, really do, but I just can't.' My voice was cracking and my eyes were filled with tears. It was ridiculous to be this upset, but I was tired, exhausted, frustrated and genuinely concerned at the fact that for the first time in my life I seemed completely incapable of getting a handle on either my own emotions or my body.

He paused, seeming to consider something while looking at me. Then his face changed. His face was no longer filled with surprise and concern. Suddenly he was stern and fierce. I knew that look. But what –

In a second he had a handful of my hair and slapped my face. It jolted me. It's the first slap in the face that usually sinks me under. There's something primal about it. Something not only physically jarring but also degrading, demeaning. In the immediate seconds after the sound cracked through the room, the silence – or was it the roar in my ears? – felt deafening, even though everything was still. We were just looking at each other, sizing each other up. My mind was still focused on the worries, but they were being pushed back as I felt the surge of adrenaline I always felt when we began this dance.

'It's not up to you when you do or don't come,' he hissed.

I glared at him. 'Seriously, you think *this* is the right time for you to become some kind of überdom? After the –'

He silenced me with a kiss, but where before it had

been sensual and passionate, now instead it was forceful, an invasion. His tongue pushed deep into my mouth, making me taste myself on him. It was embarrassing. I felt myself blush.

As he invaded my mouth he forced a hand between my legs. I tried to close my thighs, squashing his hand between them. He let out a growl of annoyance and discomfort. He broke the kiss and slapped my face again.

'Don't you fucking dare. Open your legs or I swear you'll regret it.'

The look on his face actually scared me a bit, not because I thought he would do me genuine harm, I trusted him utterly, but because he seemed genuinely annoyed. In what was surely a first in our relationship, I kept my legs resolutely shut. He gave me a long look.

'Either use your safe word or do as you are told, but stop wasting my fucking time.'

I hated the thought of disappointing him. I didn't want to use my safe word. Reluctantly I opened my legs to him and he started rubbing me roughly between my legs.

He lay down next to me and shifted me onto my side, spooning behind me in a position that would have looked innocent and intimate, but for the forearm he pressed against my throat and the barrage of filth and abuse he began whispering into my ear. The gentle kissing had, it seemed, passed.

He said humiliating and degrading things, things he knew made me wet, turned me on. He called me a whore, a slut, told me that he would tell me when I did and didn't get to come, that I had no fucking right to choose. Then came the words that filled me with terror.

'I'm going to count down to five and when I do you had better fucking come.'

I was no longer thinking about anything else, all I was focused on was the picture he was painting with his words, his hand between my legs, the numbers ringing in my ears as he counted. For a small, short while everything else buzzing around in my brain was silenced. There was just me, him, this. It consumed me.

As soon as he said 'one' it happened. I honestly didn't expect it to. I was beginning to worry about whether he would punish me for not orgasming, trying to prepare myself, when it hit me like a sledgehammer. I opened my mouth to cry out but made no noise. I went stiff for a few seconds and then started to tremble. The release was incredible. I fleetingly wondered if I might have burst a blood vessel.

I don't know if I fell asleep or was just unable to concentrate and listen, but the next thing I was aware of was Adam's voice in my ear again. This time he was soft and soothing, asking if I was OK, telling me how wonderful I was. His hand was now stroking up and down my thigh and the arm that had been round my neck was softly caressing my breast.

I turned round and buried my face in his chest, unable to look at him for a moment, just a bit overcome by it all, the pressure, the release. I thanked him, muffled against his chest, trying to hide the fact I was crying a little in relief.

He laughed softly. 'Oh, sweetheart, you don't have to thank me for anything.' He pulled the covers over us and kissed the top of my head, holding me close. His warmth felt comforting. For the first time in nearly a fortnight I felt happy and weirdly at peace. Also, bloody exhausted.

When I woke the room was still light – he must have fallen asleep when I did rather than try and disentangle himself from me to switch the light off. I couldn't tell how long I'd been asleep, but I knew it had been a while. I shifted my weight off his arm, figuring it might drop off soon if it didn't get some circulation into it.

I looked at him as he slept. He looked younger without his glasses on, oddly innocent, most definitely not the complex, occasionally stern man I had come to know. I'd never noticed how long his eyelashes were before. It made me smile. He made me smile. I felt a bit guilty, though – he'd known how to help me come when I had no idea myself how that would work, and I'd thanked him by falling asleep on him without any attempt at reciprocation. I thought it might be time to redress the balance. We had some catching up to do and, frankly, any lingering concerns about my ability to orgasm or otherwise wouldn't be an issue for what I had in mind.

Carefully I crawled down the bed. Stopping at his waist I kissed just above his groin, then either side of it. He didn't stir. I made myself comfortable on my elbows and knees, and took his soft cock between my lips, using my tongue on the underside. It began to grow in my mouth, and he began to stir, moaning softly in his sleep. I moved my mouth up and down, flicking my tongue over the tip, gently stroking his balls with my fingers.

His hand touched my thigh, making me jump a little. Keeping him in my mouth I looked round to see him smiling sleepily at me. I grinned back as well as I could with my mouth full.

His fingers began to play between my legs, sliding inside me as I took him deep in my throat. I gagged on him and it made me clench around his fingers, a chain reaction which bemused me. I began to move my mouth faster.

'Wait,' he said hoarsely.

I looked up, confused and, I'll be honest, a bit reluctant. I was having fun.

'Not this way. Fuck me.'

Oh. OK. I smiled again.

I lowered myself down on him, leaning to kiss him as our hips began moving in rhythm. Suddenly he broke the kiss, telling me to sit up. This was nothing new, he loved to watch me, to play with my breasts and see me grind against him.

As I sat up and leaned back a little he reached forward and pressed a finger between our bodies, gently massaging my clit. I moaned and began moving my hips with a little more urgency.

Then he moved his hand away and grabbed my wrist. Not hard but firmly. He moved it until my hand was near to where his had just been. He looked me in the eyes and his meaning was clear. He wanted me to play with myself while he watched.

I've done some embarrassing things for and to him, but the intimacy of it, of him watching my face so close up as I touched myself, made me feel reluctant. His gaze was unrelenting, though, his hips still while I made my choice.

It made me slightly self-conscious, but knowing how much he enjoyed watching me this way made it worth the initial awkwardness and, let's face it, when you're doing something so fundamentally fun it's no big deal really in the grand scheme of things. Also, in light of earlier, it would have been a bit churlish not to.

I started to rub my clit. He moved his hand away. He still wasn't moving his hips, but he was deep inside me and it felt amazing. I closed my eyes, focusing on how wonderful it felt and not the embarrassment of masturbating while he watched.

Then he started to talk to me. He whispered dirty things. Not humiliating, nasty things like before, but fantasies that we had shared, things that he knew turned me on. I rubbed myself a little harder and I felt another orgasm creeping up on me.

I forced myself to open my eyes and look at him. 'I'm going to come,' I said, half in amazement and half in request for permission.

He smiled and nodded at me as he suddenly started to move his pelvis up and down, fucking me hard. I watched his orgasm hit him, feeling him pulsate inside me. The feeling sent me over the edge. My thighs pressed tightly into his side as I cried out again.

After our breathing had stilled I leaned back down and kissed him. He put his arms around my neck and we lay there for a while, neither of us willing to separate just yet. And in that moment I realised what he'd done. I'd struggled to give myself an orgasm, was worried about it. While he'd been able to make me come in D/s ways, he'd wanted to show me I could still do it myself. I pressed a kiss to his collarbone. My complex, clever, lovely man.

The next morning, after the best sleep I'd had for

weeks, I lay in bed listening to his soft breathing and reflected on things a bit. Why hadn't I used my safe word? In the moment it was a complex mixture of not wanting what was happening to end, not wanting to disappoint him, and a curiosity about what would happen next. I trusted him implicitly, was intrigued (and admittedly by that point a little desperate) to see what he was going to try next. The fact that I had responded to the D/s sex in that situation when nothing else worked surprised me. It would have worried me except for the fact we had proved very quickly afterwards that it wasn't that I'd reached some kind of tipping point where the only sex I could respond to was D/s tinged – which was just as well, really, as I didn't want Adam getting flogging-related RSI or some such.

The other thing it made me realise was just how well Adam knew me, how he understood my character and personality in ways I hadn't fully appreciated until that point. A lot of the reason why he was so challenging as a dominant was, undoubtedly, because he could hazard a pretty accurate guess at any given point as to how I would react, what I would find difficult and annoying and what would come easier. But I hadn't really appreciated how he could channel that knowledge in a way that would do so much to help my wellbeing.

Since then, I've had other occasions where I've got stressed about things and found sex difficult. Our dynamic isn't such that if I feel like I'm not into sex for whatever reason, Adam gets all granite-faced and dominant and pushes his will on me anyway. Make no mistake, that's not what this was, isn't what these occasions are. There are times, when one or other of us is ill or stressed out or whatever, when things will stop for a little while. But there are other times when the world crowds in, when whatever is preying on my mind won't be shifted easily and it messes with my mojo a little. In those instances, D/s – cathartic, lovely and often vicious – can push through and clear my brain. For a little while I'm not worrying, I'm not thinking about the list of things I have to do, not prioritising whatever has to happen next, I'm just reacting. Enduring. *Enjoying*. And it's bloody lovely.

Chapter Seven

The deepening of my feelings for Adam happened quite gradually. I know I have moments when I'm a bit oblivious about emotional things, but even on that basis, I didn't expect it to be Charlotte who helped me realise the change.

Charlotte and I had met for lunch near my office. She was working nearby for a couple of weeks, and it felt like a good opportunity to catch up, albeit I knew I was going to have to deal with a fair amount of 'I-told-you-so' about the wonderousness of Adam.

I was still getting my head round the fact he and Charlotte had slept together. I knew it shouldn't bother me, knew that it was long over, knew even that he didn't want to reconnect with her and that she was happy with Tom. But somehow it felt weird. I couldn't put my finger on why. When Charlotte and Tom started sleeping together it didn't bother me that way. How could this possibly be different?

I know; even for me this was a new level of obliviousness.

Our sandwiches and coffees had just arrived when Charlotte brought up Adam and I seeing each other and how well it was going. I skirted through the conversation as delicately as I could manage.

'It's going really well. We're having loads of fun.'

Charlotte's look was all wide eyes and eyebrow waggles. I couldn't help but break into a smile.

'Lots and lots of fun,' I conceded.

She laughed. 'I knew you two would get on. You have very similar mindsets about things and obviously work together in D/s terms.' It was my turn to raise an eyebrow: this wasn't a road I was overly comfortable going down. 'And you're both quite laid-back about most things, but filthy with it.'

I nodded (she was right, after all), although it felt more difficult keeping the smile. I tried to push down this weird feeling. Was it annoyance? I didn't want to say it was jealousy because rationally I knew I had nothing to be jealous about. I guess it was more that I felt like I was still finding out things about Adam – the way he reacted to stuff, the things he enjoyed (not just the rude stuff either – he'd mentioned in passing his love of HP Sauce while we were eating lunch a week or so before, so I'd got some to keep in my kitchen) and I felt weird pangs when I realised that Charlotte might know some or indeed all of these things already. Fuck. It did sound like jealousy.

I took a bite of sandwich to try and hide my reaction. I knew it was daft. I just had to work on working through it, if that didn't sound all life-coach-tastic.

I'd missed what Charlotte had been talking about while my internal monologue had a bit of a meltdown, but my brain clicked straight back into gear as her sentence drifted into the kind of silence that seemed to inspire a response.

'So do you fancy going? The dress code isn't too formal, but you'd have to wear fetishwear.'

I had no idea what she was talking about, but I knew that anything that involved a dress code was not my sort of place, even before we got started on the outfits. I don't mind fetishwear. I find some of it hot, but I'm not the sort of person who'd feel comfortable wearing those kind of clothes out and about.

She was waiting for me to answer. Balls. I tried to prevaricate. 'Where is it again?' I paused, realising how lame I sounded. 'And, erm, when is it?'

Charlotte sighed. 'The weekend after next, at a club in the city.'

I felt vaguely relieved. I am rubbish at lying. Really rubbish. Even the simple stuff, the 'yes, Grandma, this jumper you've spent eight months knitting that isn't the right size and is made of itchy wool, fits beautifully and I love it' lies are beyond me. Thankfully I didn't have to come up with anything. 'I'm away for an old college friend's hen do that weekend unfortunately. Sorry, you'll have to go without me.'

Charlotte frowned. 'Shame. Do you know if Adam is about? Maybe he'd fancy coming with us – there's quite a group of us going. It should be a laugh.'

Adam had mentioned going to a fetish night with Charlotte previously; the conversation – when I found out they'd slept together – was one seared into my brain. He might want to go, and I wasn't going to kick up a fuss if he did – we'd agreed to be monogamous and I trusted him – but I felt massive pangs at the thought of it actually happening.

Charlotte gave me a long look, the kind of look that was way too knowing.

'You really like Adam, don't you?'

I nodded and answered, possibly too quickly. 'Yeah, of course I do. We wouldn't be doing the kind of things we do together if I didn't like him. And trust him, come to that.'

She shook her head. 'That's not what I meant, Soph, and you know it.'

I feigned confusion. Charlotte and I hadn't really ever talked deeply about emotions. I'd always given it a wide berth because with my past with Thomas it felt a bit like a weird conflict of interest – I deliberately gave them space. I gritted my teeth, wishing Charlotte had similar ideas.

'This thing with you and Adam, it's not like me and Tom, is it? It's serious. It's not just casual dating, a play arrangement?'

I stared intently at a piece of parsley garnish on my plate – honestly, who puts garnish on a sandwich? What's the point? – and tried to school my features, not blush, not reveal anything. 'Look, neither of us want the faff of anything serious. We're just having fun, nothing more.'

The awkward thing was, we both knew I was lying. Much to my relief she didn't call me on it, though. She just smirked a little. 'I knew you'd get on well together. Tom wasn't sure, but I knew.'

She sounded smug. But I let it pass. It seemed safest.

The problem with the realisation that you're in love with someone is that you have this urge to blurt it out. It's OK, I'm no Disney heroine, I'm not talking a big number with dancing animals or anything, but there were little moments when I found myself about to say it, catching myself and then stopping.

And no, I'm not just talking post-orgasm. Although, yes, that is very lovely too.

The thing was, Adam and I were fast becoming a part of each other's lives. We'd met each other's parents (mine behaved for the most part, barring an embarrassing anecdote about a school play aged six; his mum got out his old school photos and he got so embarrassed he had to leave the room). He'd come to work events with me as my plus one. I thought about him at odd moments in the day and – if the text messages and emails were anything to go by – he felt the same. He made me laugh, he was supportive, fun to be around, easy company. I missed him when he wasn't there. I was trying to be pretty laid-back about it, but the idea of disentangling our lives from each other for any reason made me feel rotten. Not, I hasten to add, that there was any reason that might happen currently, but the fact that the idea of it happening made me feel sick worried me. I know, I'm a complex woman. Or possibly a bit loopy. But the fact was, there was an Adam-sized shape slap bang in the centre of my life lately, and I loved that. Loved him, actually. But it still felt a bit precarious. Maybe my cautiousness was a weird self-defence mechanism, but I was constantly trying to divine if he felt the same way.

Of course, Adam being Adam – straightforward to the point of bluntness – he found his way to put me in the picture.

We were watching TV when I told him I loved him. I

know there's probably a whole debate to be had about whether I should have said it first, whether it was too soon, yadda yadda yadda – in fact, if my mind had been more alert at that exact moment I'd probably have had the whole debate internally before I opened my mouth.

As it was, we were sat watching the news together – him on the sofa, me on the floor by his feet, not for D/s-ish reasons, just because it was comfy to sit with my legs stretched out.

I leaned my head against him, using his thigh as a pillow, and his hand came round to my shoulder, stroking my neck, his fingers beginning to gently massage a twinge I'd got earlier in the week that had been causing me trouble (he reckoned it was from having a handbag 'the size of a small planet'. I pointed out he was an idiot, although I might then have emptied half of the contents into the bin and my desk drawer). As his fingers began to work the knot and we sat in companionable silence, I felt a surge of affection for him but also a sense that at this point there was nowhere else I would rather be in the world, and no one else I would rather be with.

Impulsively, I kissed his jeans just above his knee. 'I love you.'

His fingers kept moving and his voice behind me was languid. 'I know.'

For a split second, I felt a surge of horror. My internal monologue was beginning a panic along the lines of 'fuck, he doesn't feel the same, what does he even mean when he –' and then I stopped. My brain registered what he'd said and I burst out laughing.

I turned my head to look at him and saw him smiling down at me. As I thought. 'You arse.' His grin got wider.

'I love you too. Not least because you get my *Star Wars* references.'

I glared up at him, but we both knew it was mock fury. 'You should be so bloody lucky. Otherwise you'd have got an elbow in the ribs at best.'

He leaned down and took hold of my arms, easing me up onto the sofa next to him. He leaned down to kiss me, but before he did his face stilled just inches from mine. 'I do love you, but such empty threats are pointless.'

I stuck my tongue out at him and he leaned in, half to kiss me, half to catch my tongue between his teeth. He put his arms round me, and my hands snaked round his waist. The nibbling kiss deepened.

We didn't say anything else for a while.

Even putting sci-fi-related protestations of love aside, my relationship with Adam was unlike any I'd ever had with a guy before. He was a loving and thoughtful boyfriend, kind and caring, but also the most challenging dominant I'd ever had because of his penchant for humiliation. As a kid my mum had often repeated '*sticks and stones will break my bones, but words will never hurt me*', but Adam was the D/s opposite of that (not that I intended mentioning that to my mum, whom he had charmed in typical fashion).

Our sexual dynamic included some pain but Adam took as much if not more pleasure and amusement out of messing with my mind, not least because the better he got to know me the easier it became to tie me in knots figuratively as well as literally. But it wasn't all about the sex.

Obviously that was incredibly fun and, given half a chance, we jumped on each other at every opportunity, but I enjoyed the quiet moments, the chats between sexual she-nanigans, as much as I did the orgasms. The more we got to know each other, the more we realised we shared a sense of humour, a distaste for relationship drama, simi-lar interests, the same focus on family and friends. And the more time we spent together, the more time we wanted to spend together. Suddenly he was the person I wanted to tell if I'd had a crappy day, or drag out for payday beers. I knew he felt the same because – refreshingly – he told me. The next step was pretty much inevitable.

We'd talked about how we both wanted to get married and have kids one day (not yet, though, we were still taking precautions, although we swapped the condoms for a coil), how we wanted to live together at some point in the next couple of years, and then suddenly it happened.

His flatmate was buying a house so Adam had the option of finding new people to move into his flat or moving elsewhere. It brought our plans forward a bit but we decided to take the plunge, signing the lease on a nice two-bed flat convenient for both our offices. We were offi-cially cohabiting. Our respective parents were thrilled for us, Thomas and Charlotte were incredibly smug that their matchmaking had worked (which made them helping us move in rather irritating at points, although they were very helpful putting together our Ikea bookcases), and we, well, we were full of the joys of the honeymoon period.

Even by our standards, in between figuring out who was paying which direct debits and whose turn it was to do the washing-up, we were insatiable for the first few weeks after we moved in. We fucked in every room – although, admittedly, the flat was still on the bijou side so that only really took an afternoon – and revisited every kink and fantasy we could think of as the washing-up pile began to grow in the sink.

Actually moving in and unpacking was, unsurprisingly, slow work. We had a lot of breaks. I was on my hands and knees the first weekend we moved in, rummaging under the bed to try and make room for another box of clothes, when suddenly I felt his hands on my arse.

Before I really knew what was happening he'd pulled down my jogging bottoms – oh-so-alluring, I know – and knickers and was rubbing his hand between my legs. I stayed as still as I could, conscious that if I lifted my head up more than an inch I was going to hit it on the metal frame above me. Enjoying his ministrations, I found myself getting wet, and then suddenly his hand withdrew. I'd have felt frustrated except a second later he was pushing his cock inside me. He didn't say a word, just started moving, pounding into me as I stared at the box I'd been trying to move aside.

He slowed for a moment, and I wondered if he was going to help me up so we could fuck on the bed rather than under it, but the next thing I felt was the tip of his finger, still wet from rubbing me just a few moments before, against my arse. He slowly slid it inside me, adding it to the rhythm by pushing it in when he pulled his cock out and vice versa. I don't know if it was the surprise of the sex, the finger in my arse or the fact I was trapped under the bed but I found my excitement building quickly, and pushed back hard against his cock and finger as I came.

He withdrew from both my holes as I tried to catch my breath, and before I even realised what was happening I heard a familiar noise and the sound of a groan as he came across my arse. Then I heard him stand, zip himself up and walk away. I pulled my trousers back up – partly because I knew he'd get a kick out of it when he realised and partly out of pure necessity – and finished organising the boxes in the bedroom. When I walked into the living room a few minutes later he was sat flicking through the local freebie paper and drinking a cup of tea. A second cup sat on the coffee table waiting for me. He looked up and winked at me. I smiled back and shoved at him to make room on the sofa for me, our unpacking done for a bit.

After a few days off work to unpack and settle in together we both had to return to our respective offices. While we'd deliberately chosen a flat equidistant from our workplaces he often worked longer hours than I did so I was home at least an hour before him each night. Whichever of us made it home first tried to make it as easy for the other person as possible – starting dinner and any other necessary chores to minimise the amount of the evening taken up by household routine.

After a while, though, I hit upon giving him a more memorable – and much more rude – homecoming.

One of the major misconceptions about being submissive is that it means being passive, waiting for someone to do something to you, rather than taking the initiative. Adam had often commented on how proactive I was and how much he liked that, so, on one rather dull afternoon at work, I plotted a way to brighten his evening – albeit in a way that made me blush a bit when it came time to follow through.

Normally when he walked in the door he'd be greeted by a cheery hello, or possibly the sound of cooking or the shower depending on when I'd got in and how far into my evening routine I'd got. He'd never come home before to find me kneeling naked on the living-room floor, my mouth open, with 'please use me' written on me in that bloody red lipstick.

Trust me, it's one thing being proactive, but when your boyfriend gets turned on by filthy degrading things, it's harder to do those things to yourself than endure having them done to you. And not just logistically – finding the lipstick in his leather bag of tricks and then managing to write that across myself upside down was pretty tough. It was also difficult emotionally. My hand was shaking and I was blushing a little at the depravity of it all by the time he walked in. The theory of doing something I knew he'd find hot was one thing, but the practice of it was something different – kneeling there waiting for him to come home I began second-guessing myself, wondering whether this was a terrible idea and if actually he'd be a bit knackered after the day he'd had and rather just watch the news.

Thankfully he wasn't.

'This is a nice surprise,' he smiled, as he walked across the room. I tried not to flinch as his shoes echoed on the hard wooden floor, suddenly feeling very vulnerable as he stared at the lipstick across my chest – I knew that look was all about making me feel uncomfortable and embarrassed but I also knew that later I would be mocking him for it because it made him look like he was struggling with reading simple English.

He was a man that loved me in uniforms, underwear and all sorts of outfits, but I couldn't get enough of him in a suit. I know it's a whopping great cliché, but that doesn't mean it isn't true. The sight of him in something sharp left my throat dry. I swallowed as I watched him pull out his cock, leaving his jacket and tie on. He was good to me.

He let me lean forward and take him in my mouth, sucking him in and flicking my tongue over him.

It wasn't long before he was fully hard and, as soon as he was, I pushed myself forward, taking him down my throat and pressing my nose into his body. He groaned as I held myself in place as long as I could, eventually pulling back when I was starting to struggle for air. I watched one of his knees buckle and smiled as I suggested he sit down on the sofa.

He did so but I quickly got my mouth back around him, alternating between deep-throating him and licking the tip while using my hand on his shaft. I stared up at him, feeling myself getting wet as I looked at the pure pleasure on his face.

His quick breathing and the way he started to tense told me it wouldn't be long and I moved quickly as he curled his fingers in my hair. He let out a cry of relief as he filled my mouth. Once he was finished I put his cock away, stood up and started telling him what was in the oven for dinner as I walked into the bedroom to put some clothes on. Fear not, I got my orgasm later, but taking pleasure purely in pleasing him built the anticipation. And the one thing living together meant was that there was always time for some naughty fun.

The bigger flat and additional privacy also made for some lazy days of shenanigans with no fear of being interrupted or one of us having to go home at some point. It also meant, by dint perhaps of the amount of sex we were having and the new experiences we were sharing, that our boundaries – and my limits – began to shift.

It all started when we were curled up on the sofa on a Saturday morning watching TV together. Neither of us are morning people, and we didn't have any immediate plans so we were sat, drinking tea and watching cookery programmes and enjoying not having to be anywhere or do anything.

When he got up after his third cup of tea, I assumed he was going to the loo. At least, that was until he came back with what by now was a pretty familiar length of soft cotton rope.

Silently he took my wrists and tied them together in front of me. My heartbeat was already increasing, wondering what he had in store, but once my wrists were secure he went back to watching TV, his arm once again going over my shoulders and pulling me into him.

He stroked my hair and scratched behind my ear in a way that almost made me purr. Soon I was lying on the sofa with my head in his lap as he continued to almost absent-mindedly stroke me while we watched, somewhat surreally, a demonstration on making omelettes.

Sometimes the submissive mindset is something that comes with time, the voice in my head having to be silenced by the pleasure I feel at the things we do, but other times I can slip into it easily and deeply. Being tied up is one of the things – along with having my face slapped – that can put me into a submissive frame of mind really quickly. I was already drifting, and all he had done was stroke my ear.

We stayed like that for a long time, with him even engaging me in conversation as if this was the most normal thing in the world. I felt a little out of sorts, definitely on the back foot, but was still able to converse with him. I was even able to pick up my tea mug and drink with my hands tied in front of me. It was just like a perfectly ordinary Saturday morning, except for the fact I was conscious of how increasingly wet I was getting.

After a while he took hold of my bound wrists and lifted them over my head, leaving me feeling very vulnerable. His touch started to become more sexual as he moved his fingers up and down my body over my clothes. He gently caressed my breasts until my nipples hardened. Then he leaned down and kissed me softly on the lips and I felt like I was melting.

As the kiss deepened, his touch became rougher, mauling my breasts with one hand while holding my wrists in place easily with the other. Stretched out and held down, I had nowhere to go, and the incongruity of it – *we were watching omelettes!* – made it feel surreal. I moaned in pain and excitement.

His hand left my breast and went between my legs. He scratched along the seam of my jeans, making me shudder. He began to apply pressure, making my knickers even wetter as they were pushed against me, my clit becoming more swollen as the material was forced against it.

He rubbed firmly between my legs, through my clothes. I felt my skin get hot as he stopped kissing me and sat up, looking down at me with what seemed to be amusement. I hated it when he did that; the embarrassment felt prickly. It was as if he was mocking me. I struggled against my bindings but it was pointless, except that I felt him harden as he watched me squirm ineffectually. Git.

I thought he was going to bring me to orgasm but, when I felt myself getting close, he stopped. As I looked up at him through unfocused, confused eyes, he lifted my head, stood up and walked out of the room. I didn't really know what to do so I just stayed where I was, wondering where he had gone, what he was up to now.

Then I heard running water. Was he going to leave me in this state while he had a bath?

It must have been another ten minutes before he reappeared. He pulled me to my feet by my bindings and then untied me, telling me to quickly undress and join him in the bathroom.

I shed my clothes, leaving them on the sofa, before following him, intrigued and a little nervous, into the bathroom.

He was perched on the edge of the filled bath, still holding the rope in his hand. He told me to get in and I did as I was told, eyeing him carefully as I did so.

The water was lovely and warm and I sank into it,

thinking that I could handle most things if I got to be this comfortable. In hindsight, that was stupid and proof that I had no idea what was going on. I had underestimated him fulsomely. Still, you live and learn.

As soon as I was settled he told me to raise my hands up and he tied them again, at the wrist just as he had before.

Then he looked straight into my eyes and asked if I trusted him.

This was when the nerves set in. I'd noticed a theme with Adam, where he tended to ask this most often before he was about to do something new or fiendish to me, and wanted to be sure I was OK with it. After a moment I nodded. I did trust him, after all. I trusted him with everything.

It was just as bloody well.

Before I knew what was happening he'd placed his hand on my forehead and pushed me below the surface of the water. Our bath was one of the things I loved best about our new flat; when we'd walked round with the estate agent I had fallen in love with it – it was deep, long and claw-footed. Not that the latter mattered at this particular point, although the other two factors did. When I'd seen that bath I'd imagined us lying in it together, which we had done. I had never in a million years imagined this, though.

The splash as he pushed me under felt oddly loud to my ears, and then everything was silent except for the sound of my heart beating, the panicked thud of which filled my ears. I felt my nostrils fill with water as he held me under by the shoulders, felt my feet kick out as my instincts flared, trying to get myself up, out. After a few seconds – that felt like a fucking eternity – he pulled me back up by my tied wrists. I took in a deep lungful of air, feeling like I'd been down there for half a minute.

My long hair was soaked and stuck to my face. He brushed it away for me as I stared up at him in a mixture of awe and fear, blinking water from my eyelashes.

'Are you OK?' he asked.

My eyes held his, needing the connection, the kindness I saw there. I had never felt so powerless, so much like he had control of every aspect of me. My nose stung from inhaling the water in shock as he'd pushed me under. My breathing was ragged. But I knew I could trust him. Knew, in spite of everything, that this was something I wanted to continue. I nodded.

'Take a deep breath,' he said. I nodded again, and suddenly the world was sliding and he was pushing me under once more. This time it was for longer, maybe ten seconds or so. Maybe more. By the time he dragged me up my heart was racing and my lungs felt on fire.

He carried on for a while, alternating between pushing me under the water and leaving me to catch my breath. At one point he dunked me up and down a number of times in quick succession, leaving me gasping and water splashed across the tiled floor and his jeans. He didn't seem to mind. I couldn't help but notice that his jeans were tight across his crotch. It would seem I wasn't the only one enjoying this, despite the unusual situation.

When he was finished he told me to stand up and face the wall. With my hands bound it was surprisingly difficult to get up, and I struggled to push myself up, but he helped me. The last thing I noticed before I turned away from him was that his shirt was wet now too.

'Stick out your arse and spread your legs.'

Normally such an order would leave me feeling exposed and embarrassed – *was there a point when I'd get used to it?* – but actually I was pleased to have a moment looking away from him to regain some composure. I didn't have long to do that, though – my mistake was in assuming that he had done the most intense element of what he had planned. Definitely wishful thinking.

Out of the corner of my eye I saw him pick up a bottle of shower gel from the side of the tub and I wondered for a minute if he was going to fuck me with the curved top of it. In hindsight that might have been less humiliating than what he did do.

He washed me. He filled his hands with gel and began to rub it into my back, arse cheeks and legs. Then he rubbed his soapy hand between my legs, chuckling slightly as my legs wobbled at his intimate touch and I clutched the wall. But then came the part that made me whimper aloud in embarrassment. He rubbed up and down the crack of my arse and slid a soapy finger inside me there, half cleaning me and half finger-fucking. I closed my eyes, trying to block out the embarrassment of the assault, trying to fight the inevitable, irritating arousal it was inspiring.

When he deemed me clean he had me sit back down and washed my front, doing a very thorough job of cleaning my breasts. I'd have rolled my eyes at him for being so obvious, if I'd felt capable of looking him in the face, but by that point I couldn't quite do it.

He put some shampoo in his palm and began to wash my hair, the feeling of his fingers on my scalp making me pliant, almost sleepy under his attention. He rinsed the suds from my hair carefully, being sure to angle the shower head in such a way that he didn't get any water in my eyes and the soap ran down my back rather than into my face. His solicitousness felt surreal. He was gentle, his touch light as he helped me to my feet to rinse me down with the shower attachment until I was ready to get out (he apparently felt the need to rinse my clit for twice as long as any other part of my body). Then I did roll my eyes, but he just smiled at me, giving me his arm so I could step out of the bath.

He undid the now-wet rope from my wrists once again and wrapped me up in a fluffy, warm towel to dry me off. I curled into him as he did it and he kissed my forehead. I kissed his neck and he shivered, which made me smile against him.

When he was done towel drying my hair he told me to go back into the bedroom and lie on the bed. I did as I was told and when he entered the room he was naked, his cock hard. He climbed onto the bed and kneeled between my legs, lifting and spreading them. I blushed again as he inspected me.

He reached for the lube on the bedside table and squeezed some onto his finger, leaning forward to anoint around my arse and slowly push inside, making me gasp. Quickly he grabbed the tube again, squeezing some onto his cock, using his hand to slide it along his length.

Then he grabbed my ankles with his hands, holding my

legs upright and spread, and placed the tip of his cock against my arse. I'd had anal sex before but I'd always been bent over. Now I was looking into his eyes as he slowly inched his cock inside me.

It was humiliating, embarrassing, and insanely erotic. My previous experiences of anal sex hadn't always been positive – my tightness paired with my panic at the pain (I know, it's ironic) meant often it didn't work easily. But Adam had prepared me well: my body was ready to accept him. I put my arms round his neck as he started to fuck me – slowly sliding in and out.

I pushed my arse against him as he fucked me, urging him silently to go on, to go deeper. He whispered in my ear, telling me that I was going to come from him fucking my arse because I was a dirty little whore and it was obvious I was turned on by it. I'd had orgasms through anal play before, even anal sex, but not without an additional stimulus of some sort. That said, even as I opened my mouth to tell him I wasn't going to come that way, the orgasm hit me.

When my breathing stilled he was smiling at me with that smug look he often had. I didn't know whether to kiss him or slap him – a frequent conundrum in our sex life. Before I made my mind up he was fucking me again, a little faster and harder than before, telling me how tight I was and how much fucking my arse made him want to come too. Even before he finished the sentence he did.

Living together was brilliant. I'd been a bit concerned it was going to be strange sharing my space with someone after so long alone, but it was lovely. Adam was better than most housemates I'd ever lived with – he put stuff in the dishwasher of his own volition and was a neat freak in a way that actually worked very well for me. The one thing that took some adjusting too was, ironically, sex.

I know, it's ridiculous.

The thing is, we had a lot of sex. Lots and lots of sex. In those first heady weeks we were having sex up to two or three times a day. Before work. After work. Whole weekends. It was brilliant, exhausting, fun. We were in a cocoon of blissed-out, loved-up, sexy fun. It was ace.

Except, of course, and this is something that funnily enough no erotica heroine I'd ever heard of had mentioned, that amount of sex can bring about cystitis.

I'd never had it before and when I had my first attack I had no idea what was wrong except it hurt so much I wanted to cry. I felt comfortable sitting nowhere but the loo, although I didn't want to go even when I was there because it felt like I was weeing fire. After a few days hoping I could fend off whatever afflicted me with painkillers, a permanent hot-water bottle and force of will, I cracked and booked an appointment with the doctor. One slightly awkward conversation about how much sex I was having later and I had some sachets of cranberry-flavoured drink and (of my own volition, because I didn't fancy going to the doctors again to discuss it) cranberry pills (which I still take every day – it's just safer that way).

It wasn't the only thing that was a bit awkward to start with, despite us generally being so open with each other. The 'how do you feel about sex during my period?' convo was dealt with pretty easily – Adam was fine about it (probably more so than me, with my fears of mess), especially when he realised how frisky I got in the run up to it and thus how he'd have more chances to do ever more depraved things. Every cloud had a silver lining.

Of course, the time we worked round it by lying on the bed stroking each other to orgasm would have worked a little better if I hadn't accidentally wanked him pretty much into his own face. And then, to my shame, I got the giggles and laughed until it hurt and I couldn't breathe. His face was a picture, and then he started laughing too. By the time I'd pulled myself together enough to pass him a tissue I'd come to the conclusion that he was a keeper. Not only was he not angry but he'd seen the funny side. And sex most definitely should be fun. Although, as I pointed out to him (much) later, it was probably karma making up for the amount of times he'd wiped my juices on my own face.

These smutty and funny honeymoon-period anecdotes aren't something you can bring up with mutual friends over Sunday lunch. Let's face it, the only friends I had who might be understanding of such things (and not tempted to, at best, buy me a rubber ring for bath time and, at worst, call the police) were Thomas and Charlotte and, well, that just felt odd.

While we went out for dinner a few times together over the first months Adam and I were living together, and I spoke to and emailed both Charlotte and Thomas separately, it wasn't something I felt comfortable talking about. Firstly, that was because it was all so new that I didn't want to share it with anyone else. Secondly, if I'm honest, I still had slight pangs in the back of mind about the fact Adam and Charlotte had slept together. I know it happened before I met them, and I could hardly take the moral high ground seeing I was the only person sat round the table to have actually slept with all of them (although *that* was a revelation that made me blush when it occurred to me), but the idea of discussing the things that Adam and I had been getting up to while wondering in the back of my mind whether Adam and Charlotte had done similar things just felt strange. I knew it was irrational, and I was working hard to not let it show and get past it, not least because that kind of unreasonableness in relationships annoys me. I decided silence might be the best policy on that front for now.

Besides, from what the pair of them had told me about their relationship, I knew that what we were doing was pretty tame in comparison. It was more than enough for me to be getting on with thank you, but Thomas regaled me with tales of munches and play parties and semi-public fun that went much further than anything I had ever experienced, or would probably feel comfortable with. Thomas and Charlotte were like two adventurous kids in a playground, though, and clearly had fun together. We did, however, have one memorable night that gave a somewhat surreal insight into their shifting dynamic.

Adam and I had finally finished unpacking and invited Tom and Charlotte over for drinks and dinner to say thank you for helping us move. When they arrived Charlotte looked a bit more nervous than usual and hung back as we greeted them and ushered them into the living room. I hugged Tom hello and he and Adam shook hands. I turned to hug Charlotte, who was clutching an orchid in a pot as a house-warming gift. I took it from her, thanking them both for it (while secretly wondering how easily I could buy a replacement if need be before their next visit – I don't have the best track record with houseplants unfortunately) and then leaned forward to give her a hug. She stepped back out of my reach.

Suddenly Thomas's voice was behind me. 'She's not to hug you hello today.'

I turned to look at him, a bit confused. 'Oh. OK.'

I literally had no clue what was going on. Was she ill and worried about giving me the lurgy? Or worried *I* was ill? Did she have a bad back?

I recognised Tom's smile – previously that look would have left me feeling very nervous indeed. As it was, I was confused and definitely wondering where this was going.

'She does have something to ask you, though.'

I looked over at Charlotte. I wasn't convinced. Her lips were pressed tightly together and she didn't look like she wanted to say anything. She also had two bright points of colour in her cheeks which left me open-mouthed – in all the time I had known her I had never known her to blush. I felt Adam shifting behind me to get a better look at her, clearly equally confused.

Tom looked over at her. 'Don't you?'

Her gaze was mutinous. She nodded and closed her eyes, gathering up her courage to speak.

'Please may I kiss your feet to say hello?'

I couldn't help it, I blushed in sympathy. Fuck. This was awkward. Also, I realised to my own surprise, oddly hot.

Although maybe that was just me flashing back to some of the humiliating things she'd had me do the one time we'd played together and feeling a sense of justice. What goes around comes around.

I couldn't resist. 'Sorry?'

She was glaring at me now. I know I'm terrible to have asked her to repeat it, but, in my defence, what if I'd misheard? That'd have been embarrassing.

Her jaw was clenched, her teeth gritted. 'Please may I kiss your feet to say hello?' A pause and a quiet sigh. 'Both of you.'

Adam turned to look at me and we exchanged a slightly bemused glance. I've been intimately acquainted with feet before, but in this context it felt a bit strange. I was also a bit worried how things would escalate after this. Thomas and Charlotte remained my closest friends, but I had no interest in rekindling anything smutty with them, especially now. That said, it was definitely a kind of payback. Turns out I'm a bit of a cowbag where these things are concerned.

'Of course you can,' I smiled. In my peripheral vision I saw Adam nodding too.

I took the orchid into the kitchen and returned to find Charlotte crawling across the living-room floor towards Adam. It was a surreal sight. I felt a quickly suppressed pang of curiosity over whether this was how they had looked playing together. The sight of Adam looming over her, seeing her kneeling and pressing her lips to first one shoe and then the other, was striking. I found it oddly hot, not so much for Charlotte (although she was and remains a stunning woman) but for the view of Adam I got – the look of power, the set of his jaw, the curve of his eye-lashes as he looked down at her on the floor. It was a view that – I realised with a jolt – I didn't usually get to see because I was the one on my knees.

As I looked at them Charlotte broke the tableau and began crawling over to me. I was barefoot and suddenly very grateful I'd had a pedicure a few days before. She bowed her head and I felt her breath on my left foot, then quickly she pressed a kiss to the top. It tickled a little and I smiled, catching Adam's eyes. He and Thomas were watching intently.

She moved to my other foot and as she leaned down and pressed her mouth to my toes I heard a little sound of embarrassment, so quiet that no one else could hear it. I still had odd moments when some of the things she had done to me flashed into my mind, making me blush. But while part of me was enjoying watching her debased a little (which was mind-boggling in itself – did this count as switching tendencies?) that little whimper made me feel sorry for her. I leaned down and stroked the nape of her neck, where her haircut ended, and for a tiny moment she leaned into my caress, seemingly taking comfort from it.

The room was heavy with an atmosphere of . . . some-thing. And then just as quickly it dissipated. Charlotte got up, still blushing. I asked everyone what they wanted to drink. We decided on which takeaway to order and picked a DVD.

The rest of the evening was mostly as you'd expect. There were odd quirks. Charlotte didn't sit on the sofa next to Thomas when we watched the DVD, instead sit-ting on the floor by his feet. She whispered what I was pretty sure was a request for permission to go to the loo part way through the film. Generally she seemed a little more discombobulated than usual (Tom admitted later that he'd had her wearing a plug the whole night, which would probably have left me struggling to hold up my end of conversations too) but otherwise it was as laid-back as usual. The odd glance passed between Charlotte and Tom that made me wonder what would happen when they got home, but nothing more was said and there was no other awkwardness. By the time Charlotte kissed us goodbye as they left it felt almost normal. OK, who am I kidding? It really didn't. But as they wandered down the path hand in hand I couldn't help but feel happy for Charlotte and Tom. I don't think I'd have ever done that for my dominant in a million years, but each to their own – it seemed to be working for them.

As we closed the front door and headed back into the kitchen to begin loading the dishwasher, Adam and I simultaneously expelled a breath and then promptly laughed. I couldn't stifle my curiosity for long.

'So I have a question.'

Adam looked up from scraping leftovers into the bin. 'Go on.'

'Is that the kind of thing you did with Charlotte before? This kind of 24/7 public-ish play stuff?'

I'll freely admit I was a bit concerned – if this was something Adam was into it was a new one on me and not a path I felt ready to go down, no matter how well I knew the other people in the room with us (in fact, did knowing them make it worse? It might have made it worse).

He smiled. 'No, didn't do this kind of public play and I certainly wouldn't have had her do that in a social situation.' Phew. Although damn my stupid brain for instantly wanting to ask the obvious follow-up question – So what kind of public play *have* you done? I held back.

He broke me from my pondering. 'It was a bit of a conversation stopper, wasn't it?'

I laughed. 'It really was. I knew they were experimenting with a more intense D/s lifestyle, but I didn't realise it had got that far. Is it terrible that when Tom told her to do it my first instinct was to giggle in a kind of nervous embarrassment?'

Adam smiled. 'Me too. And I giggle horribly.'

We stood looking at each other for a moment, the silence heavy. In the end I waited until I'd turned to put a plate of leftovers in the fridge, incapable of looking him in the eye as I said it.

'Watching her do that, though, it was hot.'

When I turned back he was looking at me intently, and nodding in agreement. 'It really was hot.' He smiled. 'Especially when she kissed your feet.'

I rolled my eyes then. 'Typical bloke with your lesbian fantasies.'

He leaned over and kissed me on the nose. 'Partly. It was an interesting kind of humiliation, though.'

I shivered a little remembering it. 'It really was. Doing that in front of other people would be a hard limit for me, but that kind of level of control, of obedience . . .' I tailed off, swallowing hard to brave saying it out loud. 'I'd be curious to try it for a little while.'

Adam kissed me again. 'Just a while?'

I grinned. 'God, yes, just a while. And not too long lest you get unbearable and power-crazed.'

'It's true I do have megalomaniacal tendencies. Also, I hate micromanagement, so I probably couldn't cope for too long either.'

And that's how our foray into a weekend of full-time D/s started. I blame bloody Charlotte.

Chapter Eight

From the earliest time I'd known what D/s was, I'd been a bit dubious of the whole 24/7 thing. I've read a lot of incredibly hot fiction about it, met a few people (at my first and only ever munch and also later online) for whom I know it works really well, but I just didn't see it working for me. As ever, it's the practicalities that give me pause. What happens when he's knackered and just wants to watch the cricket, and you're waiting to be told what you can eat, or wear, or do? How does a job fit within that scenario? Friends? Each to their own and everything, but I just didn't think it would fit into my life that well.

Which isn't to say I wasn't curious.

Charlotte and Thomas's unusual visit had inspired me to try. For most of the time our evening had been completely normal, there was just an intriguing subtext. Would I want to do it all the time? No. Could I give it a go for a finite period? Would I want to? The answer was most definitely yes – particularly after our trip to the kink cottage and our blossoming relationship. I trusted Adam to be kind (ish), certainly to know my limits. And now we had our own place there was all the time and the privacy we needed to give it a go.

So we did.

The morning of the day we had decided he would have total control of me dawned like any other. It was a

Saturday. We'd had a quiet night on Friday – both of us were keen fans of the 'come home and flop on the sofa after the work week' style of Friday nights, saving more social fun for the weekend proper. In the half-doze that you have when you first wake up I had a strange feeling that the day was going to bring something important, but I couldn't immediately remember what it was. I just felt the anticipation – kind of like when you wake up and are going on holiday, or it's your birthday or something.

I rolled over to find Adam already awake and looking at me. He smiled at me and kissed me and pulled me into a nice long hug. It was lovely, loving and – in the few months we'd been living together – it was fast becoming one of my favourite ways to start the day. It was, therefore, an incongruous position from which to remind me of the rules of engagement for the day one last time.

It was pretty simple. I belonged to him completely and utterly. I had to do whatever he said, when he said it, and if I didn't there would be punishments. Every choice would be his. What I wore, what I ate, when I ate, what I did. No orgasms without his express permission either, from the moment we got up to the moment I fell asleep. Thankfully I wouldn't have to call him 'Sir' or 'Master' – we'd agreed we both felt that was a bit theatrical and would thus pull us out of the moment – but that was, essentially, what he would be.

I'd expected a bit of time before things started. Notoriously not a morning person, I was hoping I could nip to the loo and brush my teeth at least, have a moment to get my thoughts in order before we started something potentially very intense. It was a bit nerve-wracking, but the unspoken challenge of it was already calling to me – I wanted to get through the day, see where he took us. The adrenaline was already starting.

He asked if I understood what he was saying. I nodded, not trusting my voice to betray my nerves if I spoke, and worried that if he saw my fear he might somehow go easier on me, that I wouldn't get the full experience.

Ha. Chance would be a fine thing.

Tenderly he held my face, stroking my hair and looking at me intently.

'You remember what your safe word is?'

I nodded again.

He smiled. 'Good. Remember, there's no shame in using it, especially not today. I know it's going to be a big challenge for you, but I know you're going to do your best to please me.'

I looked at the man I had grown to love – smiling at me, his hair a bit rumpled from bed – and smiled back at him, knowing that he was right. Of course, it was part competitiveness as well as love that was underlying my need to do well, but I didn't think I should mention that at this point.

In hindsight I have a sneaking suspicion he already knew.

And so it began. He sent me to have a shower, while he stayed in bed reading the morning news on his phone. A product of my aforementioned morning grumpiness was that our routine had quickly formed: he went to the bathroom first, giving me an extra ten minutes in bed before I had to get up, with the handy side effect that by the time I was dressed there was usually a mug of tea and sometimes even some toast waiting for me too. So even this most innocent of initial orders felt a bit strange. Of course, things were only going to get more challenging.

Once clean and dry, I walked back into the bedroom, naked as instructed. By this point he had seen me naked hundreds of times, but as he put his phone back on the bedside table and turned to give me his full attention I felt self-conscious and embarrassed. I tried not to blush, clenching my hands into fists with the effort of not crossing my arms across my chest. I was pretty sure that would count as a no-no.

He told me to turn round, put my hands on the wall beside the bed and spread my legs apart. I did as I was told and he emerged from under the duvet to stand behind me.

His hand was at my arse, rubbing a finger cold with lube around me before sliding inside so easily I blushed a little, suddenly grateful he couldn't see my face. Then his finger was being replaced with the tip of a (very cold) butt plug that he slowly pushed all the way inside me.

His hand went between my legs and, while the touch was businesslike and almost impersonal, I couldn't stop myself from shivering, my body already signalling its pleasure at the beginning of this game, even while my brain was trying to work out whether I actually liked it.

That's not completely true. I was already – in spite of myself – railing a little under the constant orders.

He told me to turn back round. I did, silently rolling my eyes at the continuous micromanagement. Was it going to be like this all day? Because that was going to get old incredibly quickly.

I didn't school my expression quickly enough for him

not to see it as I turned. It wasn't the first time he'd seen that look on my face – and it certainly wouldn't be the last – but his reaction left me literally dumbstruck for a moment.

He grabbed a handful of my hair, holding me in place as he pushed his face next to mine. His expression was stern and his voice quiet and threatening as he warned me of how I should behave myself today.

Before I even figured out if I was supposed to acknowledge what he said with some kind of reply or whether it was safest to keep quiet he had sat down on the bed, thrown me over his lap and begun giving me a hard spanking.

As he turned my arse red I clenched against the unyielding plug. I was frustrated and turned on all at the same time, desperate to hold my own. But despite the conflicting emotions flashing through my brain (OK, I mainly felt fury), there was one incontrovertible proof of how I was really feeling about this indignity. My face was flushed and I knew I was getting wet. Damn him.

Today my arousal most definitely wasn't the point, though.

When he was finally finished I got up from his lap gingerly, my legs wobbly and my arse hot. I didn't look at him. I felt smaller. Chastened.

He got up and went to the wardrobe, leaving me standing awkwardly. He began laying clothes on the bed. Skirt. Blouse. Tie. My long stripey socks (often worn to work under my trousers, although I'd seen him eyeing them up before when I slid them on). Hair band. It would seem sexy schoolgirl was the order of the day. This should have felt comforting. I'd worn variants of this outfit for him before, even mocked him gently for the cliché. This was the Adam I knew. Loved. But still I watched him warily, knowing today the rules had changed.

Before he had me dress he wrapped a piece of rope round my waist, pulling it between my legs to hold the plug in place. He then watched as I got dressed for him. It was slow and slightly awkward going, not least because the plug and rope combination made bending to put the socks on very distracting indeed.

I know I blush a lot, but even on that basis I'm not sure I'd ever felt my face so hot without having a temperature. Finally, when I was fully dressed he had me get on my knees in front of him as he sat on the bed. Even though I was dressed and he wasn't, I still felt like the naked one.

He told me to open my mouth wide. I began to feel a little more confident – at least I could tell where this was going in the short term. He didn't tell me to suck him, though, he just grabbed my ponytail and fucked my face, hard and deep, over and over again. I gagged on him a number of times, struggling to breathe as my saliva ran down my chin, but he wasn't interested in my discomfort – he was using me as a hole to fuck, nothing more. He eventually pulled out, coming over my blouse.

He stood up and walked past with a quick stroke of my head. I clung to it as an act of tenderness because, frankly, there wasn't much else that was tender about the experience and it made me feel oddly prickly and upset. He pulled on a pair of shorts and a T-shirt and came back to stand in front of me.

'Put your coat on and go get us both some breakfast.'

I'm pretty sure I was gaping. My skirt was long enough to get away with for work if I'd been so inclined, but the socks underneath looked a little quirky.

'Where am I supposed to do that? What do you want me to get?'

I hated the nervous indecision in my voice – how quickly had that come on? – but in the light of this being his day of orders, these moments of independence seemed to take on more meaning than they would usually and I didn't want to do anything wrong. I did want to please him. My brain was also whirring at the logistics of it all. How would this even work?

His smirk as he responded seemed to indicate he too was aware of my uncharacteristic dithering. 'You decide.'

I walked to the shop. It was a bit awkward but my coat was long enough that no one had an inkling of what I was wearing underneath, and I'd wrapped a scarf round my neck to hide any evidence of the stain on my blouse. I wished I could drive to the shop, but common sense prevailed – well, that and the fact I wasn't sure I wanted to ever have to write 'wearing butt plug and crotch rope while driving' in the 'cause of accident' section of an insurance claim form.

As I walked the ten minutes to the shop I hoped the time out in the fresh air, alone, would help me regain my equilibrium, but it didn't. The plug shifted with every step, my arse cheeks were still sore from the spanking and my brain was whirring with questions about what might happen next – not least because this all felt much more challenging than I had expected, and I was desperately trying to figure out why so I could understand and hopefully move past it a little.

Unfortunately I hadn't figured it out by the time I got back home. I turned the coffee pot on and put the croissants I'd just bought in the oven to warm, still feeling uncertain about what was to come.

Once breakfast was ready Adam sat on the sofa to eat it, and gestured for me to sit on the floor between his legs.

It was strange. I often sat on the floor by choice. When I was watching TV or reading a broadsheet paper I tended to grab a cushion from the sofa and lie down on my front, stretched out to read and relax. It wasn't demeaning or any kind of status thing; it was my choice, a comfortable place to sit. But in this context it felt different, very different, and all I could remember was Charlotte sitting here a few weekends before, watching DVDs with us. Had something so simple felt this momentous for her too? This awkward?

We ate in silence, passing the jam back and forth, the TV on quietly in the background. After we'd finished eating we sipped our coffee and watched the news. He stroked my hair and I rested my head on his knee; the silence shifted subtly from feeling (to me at least) nerve-wracking to something more companionable. It suddenly clicked. The points where it felt overwhelming, oddly upsetting, were the points where there was less of an emotional connection, where he was treating me as a thing rather than a person. These moments redressed the balance, made it feel right. Even with the humiliation there was a tenderness. It was loving.

Although I had just finished my first coffee of the morning, which probably helped me feel less out of sorts too.

After the bulletin finished he told me to stand up. I did so, on slightly unsteady legs. My back still to him, he untucked my stained blouse from my skirt so he could untie the crotch rope, pulling my knickers down to my thighs so he could remove it.

He then told me to lean forward and remove the plug.

I know it's daft. He'd fucked my arse a fair few times by then, so he certainly knew what it looked like. But even so, it took a couple of deep breaths and a conscious effort to still my suddenly shaky hands before I could display myself to him that way.

As he watched me humiliate myself he reached for the lube – presumably moved from the bedroom while I was out getting breakfast. He pulled his shorts down and rubbed some onto his hardening cock. What he said next shattered the domestic feeling we'd been enjoying just moments before.

'Impale yourself on me.'

I turned my head to look at him, seeking silent clarification, though I already knew what he meant.

'Push your arse onto my cock.'

He was sat on the sofa. It wasn't especially low, but lowering myself down on him was awkward and took some manoeuvring to ensure I didn't squash him, but was able to get him inside. His groan of pleasure as I settled myself onto his lap filled me with pride. My head rolled back, resting on his shoulder as I enjoyed the feeling of him deep inside me.

After a few moments I began to move, slowly, my feet on the floor helping give me leverage to move up and down. The movement against made my arse, which was still smarting after my spanking, hurt. It was also humiliating: effectively I was giving him my arse while he sat there. But it was also incredibly hot, even before his hand snaked round to my clit.

I hadn't come earlier, so was already somewhat overwrought, even before he began rubbing me, making me writhe harder against him.

My orgasm built quickly, and it was only at the last second that the voice in the back of my head reminded that I should ask for permission before I came. My thighs were shaking with the effort of staving it off as I grudgingly pushed the words out, although he had me repeat them before he finally took pity on me and let me come, loudly and with such force that it was only him grabbing my waist that stopped me toppling off the sofa.

As I came back down to earth he stroked my hair, kissed my neck and whispered that he was pleased I was being such a good fucktoy, something that in another mood might have left me glaring at him, but instead made me grin in adrenaline-fuelled glee. I turned to look at him and, impulsively, he leaned forward and kissed me deeply.

'You look so beautiful, all dishevelled and covered in filth.'

I restrained the urge to stick my tongue out at him (I knew *that* wasn't going to go down well today) and instead kissed him back, enjoying the moment of tenderness.

One of the interesting things about moving in together was the way we complemented each other. I was organised, always had been, partly because of work and partly because I'd spent so many years living alone whereby if I didn't sort myself out then no one else would. Adam, on the other hand, loved the fact that I sorted out a lot of the admin born of us moving in together, and instead picked up the slack with something I've never really been overly fond of. Cleaning.

I know living in a clean and tidy house is a wonderful thing, but I have to say I am not a natural cleaner. Every so often I'll have a blitz, if someone is visiting or if it reaches that tipping point where suddenly it feels like you couldn't possibly live like this for a moment longer and must act immediately (see also: eyebrow growth – how is it I can go to bed looking vaguely OK and wake up looking like the mono-browed missing evolutionary link?). Adam, on the other hand, loved cleaning. The first thing he did when we moved in together, while I was alphabetising our DVD collection (don't judge me) was to arrange our kitchen. A fun Saturday morning for him started with him scrubbing the bathroom till it gleamed while I bought the papers and made breakfast. He enjoyed it, seemed to get a lot of satisfaction from it, and it was one of the (many) reasons why I thanked my lucky stars I'd fallen in love with someone as wonderful as him.

Not today, though.

Today he just seemed keen to test me. He sat on the sofa and had me clean the living room around him. I dusted, polished and vacuumed, with him barely lifting his legs out of the way as necessary, the whole time aware that he was watching me and looking up my skirt as I bent over.

Still, if this was what he had in mind for his day of total control who was I to quibble?

When I was done he walked around, inspecting my work. It was a better job than I'd usually have done under my own steam, but he was meticulous – or possibly looking for excuses.

He found a patch of dust at the back of the DVD player, and wiped his hand across it to hold it up to me. My face wrinkled as I stared at the – frankly barely noticeable – grime on his fingertips. I grabbed my duster and leaned down to push my arm right into the TV cabinet to reach it, barely aware of myself harrumphing 'for fuck's sake' under my breath.

He cleared the distance between us in seconds. He didn't even look at me but just grabbed my arm as he walked past me, dragging me with him. I was barely aware of what was happening, he moved with such speed.

He opened a door in the corner of our living room to reveal our small storage cupboard. When we'd moved in we'd put empty boxes that needed disposing of in there as we'd unpacked and my first thought when he opened the door was, 'Oh, he's cleaned it out and taken all that stuff to the tip.' Until he pushed me inside and down to the floor and closed the door, leaving me in the dark and mostly empty (there was a throw we used on the sofa when it was cold but that was it) cupboard.

It all happened so quickly that I was stunned for the first few minutes. I sat, cursing him under my breath (quieter than I had moments before), waiting to see what would happen next. What the fuck was he playing at? I felt furious more than anything else. I knew I'd agreed to the terms of engagement but what the fuck was this? Part of me wanted to open the door, but several things stopped me – curiosity at what he was going to do, and pride that refused to let him see that he was bothering me or that this was upsetting me. I thought about opening the door, moving out and seeing what would happen but since I didn't want to apologise and had no intention of safe-wording the only thing likely to happen would be that I'd get myself in more trouble. Bad plan.

I waited, as patiently as I was able (which wasn't very).

The only light in the room came from under the door. I watched as it flickered at points, wondering if that was him walking past. I strained to hear if he was outside, and was unsure whether I would be relieved or nervous if he was. Through it all, though, I seethed. I felt proper, burning fury of the kind I had felt in D/s situations before, but never with Adam.

I don't know how long I sat there, but over time I began to soften. I stopped feeling angry and began to feel anxious. I felt bad that I might have disappointed him or let him down, annoyed with myself that these seemingly simple orders had proven so challenging – confused, if I'm honest as to why they had felt so tough. I lay down and curled myself into a ball as I waited for him to come back.

Finally he opened the door and beckoned me out. I tried to get to my feet but he told me to stay on my hands and knees. I peeked at his face as he moved past me and tried to read his expression, but for the first time I really couldn't.

I crawled behind him as he walked across the room. He stood by the entertainment unit that housed our TV, games console and DVD player, then finally turned to look at me, unzipping his shorts as he did. I automatically opened my mouth but he grinned – a brief but reassuring return of my Adam – and shook his head.

He stroked himself while I watched. I'd seen him do this before, but whereas normally it felt acceptable to help him along, this time I knew I could only watch. It was an erotic kind of torture, especially as he began to move faster, getting ever closer to coming.

Finally he groaned and aimed his cock down. For a split second I thought he was aiming for another part of my body or outfit, but instead he came on the wooden floor.

He told me later that the look on my face at that moment was a picture of confusion and annoyance. I can't imagine it got any better when he spoke to me – I literally had to restrain the urge to push him over.

'This is why, when I say clean the room, everything has to be clean. Now lick it up.'

I looked up at him, trying to work out if he was serious or if this was some kind of head fuck. I knew him well enough by then that I could tell that he wasn't messing with me, that he was unmoved by my pleading glances. I think he knew me well enough by then, though, to know that I wasn't going to safe word my way out of it.

Slowly I bent down and licked at his cum, tentatively, but it just moved across the wooden surface away from me. Bloody laminate floors. I moved to try and catch it on my tongue, aware it was a ridiculous and surprisingly difficult quest. It took ages, and by the time I'd finished my eyes were teary with humiliation. I also felt like I'd disappointed him and let him down. It was a weird, unexpected feeling that made me want to howl. It caught me off guard. He saw it for what it was, though.

As soon as he saw my face he picked me up off the floor and took me to the sofa. We sat down together, he held me in his arms and hugged me and I clung to him, in a way that afterwards I would feel a bit sheepish about but which at the time felt so desperately important. I needed the connection, I needed his warmth. I needed him.

His voice was calm, gentle. He told me I'd done well, that he was proud of me. He asked me if it was OK, if he had gone too far.

After the initial reaction to the humiliation of it all I calmed a little. He grabbed the throw from the cupboard and wrapped it round me, pressing a soft kiss to my lips before disappearing to make two mugs of tea.

As I drank the tea I began to feel slightly less bereft. I'd had intense D/s experiences before – more humiliating things, definitely more painful things – that had affected me much less. We quietly talked it through, what we had found hot, what I had found difficult, and why.

Bearing in mind how articulate I can be about some elements of my mindset, on this one I was a bit stumped. I've been treated impersonally before, I've been hurt before, I've been humiliated in other, similar ways. I don't know if it was the fact this had happened within our home environment that made it feel somehow more intense; I don't know if it was being shut in the cupboard – it's definitely possible. In hindsight I wonder if it was the sense of being properly punished for a misdemeanour, rather than it being 'play' punishment, that pushed me over the edge.

Whatever it was, slowly I began to feel more myself

again. We drank our tea, and I had a restorative chocolate Hobnob (I think the sugar helped lift my mood too – that's my excuse and I'm sticking with it) and as we cuddled on the sofa my mindset shifted once more.

We still had a whole afternoon set aside for smutty fun, and while by, unspoken agreement, Adam's time in control had come to an end I was still feeling frisky and wanted to show my appreciation of him, his kindness and understanding. So I set about doing so in the filthiest ways possible. I lay in his lap licking and sucking him gently while we watched the rugby, enjoying half-teasing, half-worshipping him for the entirety of the game. Then I asked, of my own volition and with way less of an angry expression, if he would let me suck him until he came, touching myself while I did so. Then I gave him the filthiest kind of show, the kind of thing that made me blush but always made his eyes darken with lust.

It was stuff that in a different context was humiliating, that I would have felt prickly over if he'd made me do it. But I wanted to do it by choice. It made me wet to do it for him, to see how hard it made him.

My humiliations had felt almost too much to bear, but doing the same things voluntarily felt OK.

I know, I'm a contrary woman. Some kinksters would undoubtedly say that my behaviour was a poor show on the submissive front, and maybe it was. But between us we discovered our limits and figured, without a shadow of a doubt, that 24/7 type control wasn't for us. Although, as Adam admitted while we were brushing our teeth that night, that wasn't a bad thing.

'Some days, Soph, it's all I can do to sort myself out

through the day, much less micromanaging you. It just didn't feel natural to me. I want an equal partner that submits, not a slave that obeys. Giving you real punishments didn't excite me the way other play did. It just made me feel like a bit of a dick.'

I laughed as I gargled.

'I know that probably bars me from the Dom club, but then I never really read the rules of entry, and would have probably ignored them anyway. It's like the Groucho Marx quote – "I don't want to belong to any club that will accept me as a member."'

I sighed with relief. Thank fuck. He kissed me on the ear.

'Shall we just keep doing what works for us? That means you can mock me without wondering if I'll get all po-faced and make you apologise for a lack of respect. We can do D/s stuff, or normal stuff. Or just watch telly and eat toast. That's pretty much my idea of an ideal relationship.'

He was right. And it saved us from having to sort out a blimmin' sex contract.

Chapter Nine

I am not a bratty sort, although I suppose bratty sorts would probably say that too. At times, though, I can be somewhat . . . exuberant, shall we say. Cheeky even. With Adam it was fine, for the most part, because our relationship was based on a D/s dynamic that wasn't po-faced. He was secure in his dominance of me without me having to call him Lord Farquhar Master of All, curtsey or refer to myself in the third person. The dynamic between us ebbed and flowed depending on what we were doing, where we were and who was around. Sometimes the banter between us got very impudent, and even silly. In the right mood, if he remembered, later he might exercise mock retribution for my 'misdemeanour', but as he loved to tell me, he didn't need a reason to 'punish' me: when the time came and if he felt the urge he would just hurt me because we both enjoyed it. That was all the justification he needed.

He wasn't wrong.

There was no sense of me being 'punished' for being me. Mostly he let me get away with any minor mocking, seeing it as a sign of affection, which is what it was, and was generally tolerant of my smart mouth, which even my submissive tendencies can't keep in line.

Well, mostly tolerant.

I will admit I'd been mocking him more than usual,

although if you asked me I'd be hard-pressed to tell you why. I was in an especially good mood, which probably exacerbated it as when I'm happy I tend to be quite irreverent. It was in the aftermath of a particularly heavy scene we had done a few days before, which was playing on my mind – in the positive, flashbacks-popping-in-your-head-to-make-you-flush-with-arousal-and-shame-while-waiting-for-the-kettle-to-boil sort of way. Perhaps it subconsciously inspired me to rebel a little more than usual as a way of reasserting my equilibrium in the face of my memories of lying on the kitchen floor naked, bruised and covered in his spunk. Mostly, though, it was because we had company in the form of some old university friends of mine who came to visit for the weekend and who were blissfully ignorant of what we got up to in the bedroom.

So I pushed. Whenever my university friends get together the mocking and sarcasm flows, and it was easy to get caught up in it. And it was funny to see his eyes narrow as he looked at me as everyone laughed, his eyes saying, 'If they weren't here you'd be bent over the sofa right now being made to feel very sorry for what you just said,' as mine sparkled back at him pretty much saying, 'I know, but they are. Ha!'

In hindsight, I pushed too far. It didn't feel it at the time, though. As we made dinner – dim sum from the Chinese supermarket, followed by stir-fried beef with ginger and spring onions, washed down with cold beer – the banter continued. I saw his eyes narrow at the cheekiest of my comments, but knew that he could do nothing about it. It really made me smile, and the humour in his replies and the way his tactile tendencies continued unabated left me fairly sure he was taking it in good spirits. And to be fair, he did – his smile was indulgent, his eyes twinkling.

As we were loading the dishwasher, our guests in the living room setting up the Scrabble board, he pulled me over for a kiss. Laughing, I hugged him, caught up in the fun of the day, loving how well he was getting on with my friends, just enjoying good company and a lovely time. Our kiss deepened and suddenly we were staring at each other with that look of two folk who – no matter how friendly the company – just want to rip each other's clothes off.

I could read the lust in his eyes, and I was pretty sure mine mirrored his. Suddenly Scrabble wasn't the game I wanted to play. I leaned up to kiss him again, nipping his bottom lip with my teeth. He growled at me.

'What is it with you today? You're in a very hyper mood.'

I grinned at him around his lip. 'Sorry. I can't help it. I find it funny doing these things while other people are around.' I pinched his arse. Quite hard. He winced. 'Don't look like that, you big baby. You do worse to me. It's just you have a low pain threshold.'

He looked with mock outrage. 'Baby? Me? Wait till we're alone, then we'll see who's a baby.'

I grinned at him, pinching his arse again as I pressed a kiss to his nose. 'Good comeback. Talk is cheap. There's nothing you can do until Sam and Emily have gone home. Too noisy.' I pulled a face of mock upset. 'Oh well . . .'

He grabbed my shoulders and pulled me in for another kiss. 'Oh my lovely, foolhardy Sophie.' He leaned in to whisper in my ear. I tried not to shiver. 'Challenge

174

accepted.' He nipped my earlobe with his teeth and before I could really react or the words had sunk in, he'd picked up the bottle of wine and walked through into the living room, whistling.

Just when I thought the day couldn't get any more fun, the game was on. And not just Scrabble.

I'd showered before bed to try and minimise pressure on the bathroom as we all got ready in the morning, and came into the bedroom damp and wearing just a towel. He was waiting as I pulled the door closed and before I realised what was happening the towel had been yanked off me and thrown to the floor, the cool air bringing goosebumps to my damp skin. His hand tangled in my hair and dragged me across to the bed. I yelped in surprise and his hand went over my mouth, silencing me.

In the mirror on the opposite wall my eyes looked wide, shocked and a little nervous, although they shone with anticipation – even the worst nerves never managed to shake the anticipation. He smiled at me, but his expression was a little dangerous as he leaned down, his breath whispering warmly against my ear.

'Keep very quiet now, do you understand?'

I nodded, but his hand tangled tighter in my hair mid-movement and held me in place. My heart began to beat a little faster. The shutters were down; my playful boyfriend had given way to my strict dominant. The anticipation, the sense of challenge, began to build. He was looking at me expectantly and, now more than ever, I knew it was important to respond. I made a hopefully vaguely affirmative grumble from the back of my throat.

He didn't speak again as he manoeuvred me onto the bed. The duvet had been moved aside ready for my arrival, and the cuffs were already looped round the frame. Before I knew it, my wrists and ankles were secured with the heavy-duty cuffs that he usually ignored in favour of elaborately wound rope. This meant two things: he didn't intend to waste any time with prettiness, and he intended to do something he didn't want me wriggling free from. My nerves were rising, even before he turned round to check a pile of things which I couldn't quite see on his bedside table.

He lay down next to me on his side, using his hand as a headrest. For long moments he didn't speak, instead just looking at me stretched out and vulnerable, his gaze hungry, assessing. I tried not to move, tried to keep his gaze, tried to do everything I could to not betray how nervous I was – and already how wet. To be honest, bearing in mind how well he knew me and how stretched out and open I was, I don't know how much luck I had with either, but a girl has to try, right?

Right.

He brushed a stray strand of hair away from my face and began to whisper to me.

'I love your quick-wittedness and your wicked sense of humour, you know that. I love the fact that we fit together so well, we challenge each other.' I nodded, my polite acknowledgement seeming somewhat incongruous under the circumstances. 'But sometimes I think you're a bit foolhardy. Pushing me because you thought there were no consequences, because with the house full you thought there was no chance of me doing anything with you.'

I swallowed hard, my heart beginning to pound. 'You were a bit rash there, weren't you?'

I opened my mouth to argue, saw the look in his eye and decided some kind of self-preservation was in order, especially since we both knew he was right. Not trusting my voice, I nodded again, albeit more slowly this time.

His chuckle sounded loud as he shook his head at me, grinning. 'You should never underestimate my creativity.' A pause. 'I can come up with ways to punish you if I want to.' He leaned down to kiss me, and I arched up, trying to deepen the kiss. 'Not that I need an excuse, do I?'

I shook my head, smiling shyly.

He kissed me softly again, stroking my hair out of my eyes. 'Oh, sweetheart, that's probably for the best.'

Even with the anticipation, the nerves and his stern gaze I still felt a swell of love for him. And then he moved, and the nerves burst back to the fore.

In hindsight my complacency seems like lunacy. Even then, in the back of my mind, I didn't expect whatever he was going to do to me to be especially challenging. How could it be? Logistically? He'd hurt me before and while at its most harsh it had been difficult to bear I'd got through it all in the end, mostly unscathed and quiet. What could he do now, with people in the next room, that could be worse than the flogger, or the crop, or the worst of his humiliations?

Ha. Foolish me.

He started with the pegs. Eyeing them cautiously as he lined them up beside me, I counted ten. This didn't look good.

Straight from the washing basket, the pegs were wooden, vicious and unyielding, and I sucked air desperately into my lungs as the pain began to thrum through my nipples when, in businesslike fashion, he clamped them both.

Whatever he was doing, he didn't intend to hang around. My chest was still heaving with the desperate gulps of air as I processed those first few moments of pain. Then he moved down my body with another a peg, his fingers sliding along my cunt lips. In a split second I realised what he intended to do. I sat bolt upright, or tried to at least, my head jolting up, my arms and feet, which were still caught by the leather cuffs, pulling urgently but ineffectively.

'Adam, no, don't do –' I trailed off, mindful of his earlier order of quiet, and aware of his glare at my panicky voice. He moved away, shaking his head at my impertinence, but any relief I had at him having stepped away from his prize vanished when he came back with the ball gag, which was shoved unceremoniously into my mouth and tightened up around my head. He picked up the peg again and, giving me an evil smile, slid his finger into my cunt, separating me so he could put the peg directly on the flesh of one of my lips.

To my embarrassment I was so wet that to start with it slid off. He chuckled quietly, and I glared at him. He tutted, wiping a finger along my face in warning, and then went back to try again. He managed to slide it on and it clipped in place. The sharp pinch made me whimper, and I breathed in deeply through my nose to try and process the pain.

Moving quickly, he added another peg next to the first, and then two more on my other lip. I was starting to struggle a little, although of course I had nowhere to go. I focused on trying to stay still. On letting the pain wash over me, acclimatising to it. Welcoming it almost. I also had a strong sense of not wanting him to see how much he was getting to me. Forget my competitiveness at Scrabble, this was on a whole different level, and he knew it. Suddenly he was putting pegs on my ears, one on each lobe. The ridiculousness of it (and also the pinch) roused me from my trance, and I glared at him again. He smiled, and I felt my gaze soften in spite of myself, loving the game even while I was trying to beat him at it. I know technically it's pretty much impossible for me to 'win' within our dynamic but that wasn't going to stop me trying, wide-eyed optimist that I am. Or idiot. Either or.

He leaned down and kissed the ball that was settled within my mouth.

'Just two more.'

Two? Seriously? I only saw one. Hmmmmm.

He ran his finger along my bottom lip, grabbing it and pulling it away from the gag, for another bloody peg. I was shivering a little by then. The pain was unexpected but the main thing I felt was humiliation. It's daft, I know – he'd done much meaner things to me in the past, but being immobile and treated this way made me feel so much at the mercy of his whims. It also made me incredibly wet, and that paradox – the tiny voice in my head asking 'How can this be hot?' – made me flush more, not least because as he held up the final peg I could pretty much put money on where it was going to go. Lucky number ten.

He put it on my clit, and the touch of his fingers between my legs made me shake with a mixture of anticipation and arousal. I could see his erection in his trousers; he was getting off on this as much as I was.

He knew me well, his eyes noticing the direction of my gaze.

'Oh, sweetheart. Do you want me to fuck you?'

I nodded, aware I was eager – too eager, perhaps – but beyond caring. He smiled at me.

'One last thing and then you'll be ready.'

I wasn't really sure what he was doing, just that he was lifting my arse off the bed with his hands at my hips. Suddenly something was pressing to my arsehole, sliding in a little way and then stopping. Way too small to be a plug, but something with a ridge to it that meant it only went in so far and then –

What WAS that?

He stood up from the bed and waved at me. 'Just going to wash my hands. Don't want to rub it somewhere painful.'

He told me afterwards my face was a picture. I literally had no idea what he had done, and my mind was spinning.

My arse was tingling a little bit. It was an odd feeling but not unpleasant. Kind of warm. I clenched my arse, tightening around whatever it was he had put there, trying to feel what it was, and suddenly the tingling felt hot in a way that was less pleasant. What the fuck was it?

When he came back and settled himself on the bed he put me out of my misery. 'Ginger. I decided to save you a piece while I was preparing dinner.'

A small part of me saluted his organisation. The rest, feeling the increasing heat in my arse, would have kicked him if my legs were free.

I'd heard of figging before – the practice of putting a small hand-carved plug of fresh ginger in a submissive's arse. I'd not experienced it, though. On top of the sensations of the pegs all over my body, it was feeling very intense, and that was before Adam slowly pulled open the pegs between my legs and pushed himself inside me.

He slid in easily, groaning appreciatively as I opened myself eagerly for him in spite of myself.

He began to move, pushing the ginger deeper inside me as he did so. Every thrust seemed to knock one peg or another and the bursts of pleasure and pain of his movements left me unable to do anything other than react to whichever came next. Eventually they mingled together, and I began whimpering behind the gag, enjoying the anachronism of the two extremes of feeling.

He came after a few minutes, a product I think of the knowledge of his power, paired with my increasingly frenetic squirming underneath him as the ginger increased in intensity. It was beginning to burn a little, and I found myself shifting my arse, although if you'd asked me if I was trying to manoeuvre it out or rub at the pain I wouldn't have been able to tell you. He pulled out and stood up, walking across the room to grab his belt.

My eyes must have widened because he smiled at me and stroked my face; it was a mockery of reassurance.

'Don't worry Soph, I'm not going to hit you with the belt – not tonight anyway.' I felt relief, tinged with a weird kind of disappointment – even with the range of different sensations he was inflicting upon me I was still pathetically eager for more. 'I think you're going to start squirming more shortly, so this is going to help keep you still.'

I watched warily as he picked up the expanding butt plug I'd bought but discarded as too large for my arse. Picking delicately between the pegs he opened me up and pushed the plug inside me. Shit. I could see where this was going. The bulb hissed, expanding the plug inside me. I couldn't help it, I moaned. He pressed it again, filling me up. Then he leaned down and tied his belt around my thighs, tying them together to ensure I wasn't (accidentally or otherwise) going to push the plug out.

Then he switched it on.

At that point the fact I was tied down was probably for the best, as otherwise I'd have surged off the bed. The vibrations in my cunt were causing me to writhe, which had knock-on effects on both the ginger plug and the pegs. Every tiny movement, every breath even, had an impact, a consequence of pain or pleasure.

I burned.

The feeling in my arse was getting increasingly intense. He lay down next to me, resting his chin on his arm, watching intently. If I could have moved I think I'd have definitely kicked him now. I felt like a specimen in an experiment.

I didn't want to move, but I was finding the ginger in my arse increasingly painful. The cacophony of pain from across my body was shifting as suddenly the feeling of the burning sensation overtook everything else. My eyes began to water, and I began to whimper desperately behind my gag.

Adam smiled.

'The thing about ginger is it takes a little while to warm up. I think you're probably getting close to its maximum potency now.'

Getting close? I wasn't sure I could cope with anything more. He laughed softly, which makes me think my incredulity was written on my face.

'Don't worry, the pain will begin to ease. In about another ten minutes or so it'll be just like you've got an ordinary plug in your arse – although one significantly smaller than usual.'

I blushed.

'It might hurt more before it gets better, though. But don't worry, sweetheart, I'll be here with you the whole way.'

And that he was. He played with me, like a cat playing with a mouse. He watched the agony play across my face as the ginger sting turned into a full and fierce burn, watching my eyes begin to water. He watched me try and control my breathing to work through the pain and, when I'd done a good enough job that my obvious distress began to subside, he unclipped and then re-clipped a peg on my nipple. The release and then reapplication of the pressure pushed through my calm and began a whole new wave of pleasure. He stroked my hair, ran his fingers along my face, kissed the top of my breasts. He told me how proud he was of me, how brave I was, how hot it was to watch me endure for him, with his cum drying on my thighs, what a filthy whore I was for not only letting him do these things to me but for getting off on them.

And he was right, I was. The pain was blurring together, merging with the relentless vibrations between my legs.

I was being buffeted around in a sea of sensations, aware of nothing but the pain and his voice whispering in my ear, grounding me, telling me I could do this, I could withstand this.

Then he began removing the pegs and I really wasn't sure that I could. The strange thing about being clamped is that after a while you can't feel it much any more. Once something has been pressed for so long that it's gone a bit numb it stops being an aggressive pain, mellowing to a dull ache. My body was a mixture of these aches, until Adam began unclipping the pegs. He started with the ones at my mouth and my ears, gently rubbing life back into them to minimise the pain as the blood began to flow again. Then he moved to my breasts and unclipped those. He didn't rub my nipples, though. Tears began flowing freely then, the pain rising until I was splashing tears on my poor punished breasts. Eventually he took pity on me, kissing both nipples softly, taking them in his mouth one at a time, soothing them gently with his tongue.

As he moved down my body I began to shake. I had no sense of time passing, but surely the ginger burn should be calming down by now? As it was, I was continually whimpering behind my gag, unable to control my reactions, thankful that he *had* gagged me because otherwise I would have been howling by this point. His hand went between my legs. I couldn't decide if I was thankful or annoyed that he took the pegs on my lips off so quickly. The burst of pain was intense enough that I saw stars, but at least it was over quickly, and his hand rubbing between my legs was a very welcome change of pace.

Finally I was left with one peg on my clit, the ginger in

my arse and the too-big-plug vibrating away in my cunt. He stopped for a moment, looking down at me again, drinking in the sight of me. Then, to my rising panic, he pressed the bulb on the plug once more, filling me utterly, and changed the speed of the vibrations inside me. Suddenly my moans were the inevitable precursor to an orgasm that I was a little worried might knock me off the bed. Maybe it was just as well I was tied down.

He leaned in, kissing my cheek where a track of tears was drying.

'Are you going to come for me now, my brave, good girl?'

I nodded, although to be honest I wasn't sure if I would be able to overcome the whirl of sensations enough to lose myself in orgasm. Sometimes, though, he knows what my reactions will be in such situations better than I know them myself.

He unclipped the peg at my clit and began rubbing it with his fingers, both to mitigate the pain and increase the pleasure. I felt myself begin to slide under, looking to him, watching the nod and the smile on his face as I surrendered myself to the sensation.

I came so hard it hurt. In the immediate aftermath I was disconnected from what was going on, my breathing loud and my limbs loose as he moved around me, taking off the cuffs, rubbing my arms, pulling out the gag and then, finally, reaching round and pulling out the piece of ginger.

He wrapped it in a tissue and threw it in the bin, washing his hands again before climbing back in bed with me. I was quiet, replete. After the most intense submissive experiences it takes a little while for me to come back to earth. I was a slightly dazed and almost sleepy version of myself.

He cuddled me close, and I curled into his body heat gratefully, seeking that connection and closeness as I began to resurface. He kissed my hair and stroked my back and I clung to him, a little overcome. Speechless.

'See? Creativity. I don't need to worry about noise.'

It took a few seconds for me to understand his words, and when I did I laughed to myself, suddenly mindful of the game that had started all this.

'You're definitely right. Is that what you want to hear? You're right.'

He grinned at me. 'Come on, Soph, when don't I want to hear you tell me I'm right?'

I stuck my tongue out at him. 'That was incredible, though. The ginger hurt so much, but the increase in intensity was amazing. Moving from the tingle to the burn, until the point where it was all I could do to cope with the pain.'

He nipped my earlobe with his teeth. 'It was fucking hot to watch. I do like making you squirm.'

I nodded solemnly. 'That you do.'

He grinned at me. 'Next time we do it I'm going to have you on all fours and spank and then flog you as you begin to squirm.'

Maybe it was because, whilst the pain had burned fiercely, it ended almost as soon as the ginger was removed, but my first thought was one of anticipation.

'I can't wait.'

'I know. Minx.'

I switched off the light and we went to sleep, him secure in the knowledge he'd been proved right, and me not giving a toss about that but feeling the lovely after-effects of the satisfaction and release of a wonderfully intense evening.

Was it terrible I was plotting ways to badger him the following day to see what he'd do to top it? Maybe I *am* a brat.

Chapter Ten

Ginger was just one of many new experiences Adam introduced me too. Another I enjoyed, much to my surprise, was watching porn together. Before I met him my knowledge of porn was born mostly of prejudice and those fifteen-minute free previews you get on hotel pay-per-view channels, mostly of fake-breasted women with false fingernails. I know, fingernail extensions are a daft thing to get irate about, but I found them ridiculous – who could believe these women could happily wank when they had talons so sharp it was like watching Wolverine masturbating? I know, probably the average porn film maker isn't worrying about my preoccupation with Stanislavski's willing suspension of disbelief, but it mattered to me.

I'm definitely no kind of prude, but my choice of erotic inspiration was always text-based, from my earliest forays into buying Black Lace books and reading Literotica online. When Adam first mentioned us watching porn together I rolled my eyes. I just wasn't interested. I'd rather have had sex watching the Test Match Special, and that really didn't float my boat either. But one night, curled up in bed, he showed me a bit of a scene involving a beautiful (but not fake-looking) brunette woman with amazing eyes. The D/s element was minimal, it was beautifully shot and not too – for want of a better word – gynaecological.

It felt real and by the time he reached between my legs my enjoyment was, not to put too much of a fine point on it, obvious. I later learned the woman's name was Stoya. Adam showed me another couple of films he had with her in them, then together we found some other films with hot, real-looking women who reacted like normal women would having sex (no claws and no shrieking orgasms of the sort that made me raise an eyebrow in his direction). My favourites, along with Stoya, were Madison Young, Sasha Grey and the Australian domme Chanta Rose. The thing about all these women is that they completely went against my preconceptions of what women working in porn were like. Articulate, sexually liberated (and certainly not being taken advantage of by anyone), intelligent, creative – the kind of women I'd love to go for drinks with because they seemed interesting and like they had something to say.

Over a period of time we watched a fair few scenes curled up together in bed, and I became a convert. We didn't watch it every time we had sex – I think doing anything *every time* you have sex together is a bit of a concern – but as part of our sexual repertoire it was fun. It also provided a springboard to lots of discussions about what we were into and what we might like to try. The porn itself varied from being quite straightforward sex (including a Batman parody that managed to be both hot and hilarious) to very intense D/s type scenes which made my throat dry. But as much as I loved those, I also loved the scenes of aftercare, where the submissives who had been involved in the action bundled up in bathrobes, their faces showing the same euphoric endorphin-laden smiley reactions I did after something intense but hot. I could relate to them. I believed them. And the fact this porn was something aimed at me rather than just blokes appealed. A lot.

As for Adam, he loved how much I enjoyed it and that it was something we could share. I think he also approved of the fact we could have conversations about attractive women without me being funny about it. I was definitely secure in our relationship and where we were at – I don't look like a porn star (although from what I can tell, away from the cameras most porn stars don't look like porn stars either), and Adam wasn't expecting me to look like one any more than I was expecting him to look like either James Deen (a prolific and increasingly mainstream male porn star) or Damian Lewis (it's something about his eyes).

I know for some people porn is a major taboo, but with Adam I found that the better I got to know him and the more I trusted him, the happier I was to experience new things. I was deeply in love with him, I knew that he loved me and I trusted him to protect me. I'd trusted the previous dominants I'd played with to a lesser extent, but the more intense experiences we had together, the better we could read each other. I trusted him to know what I could cope with and what I couldn't, to know what my reactions meant in any given situation.

Of course, sometimes he used this knowledge to mess with my mind in evil ways – not least because he knew I am both impatient and incredibly curious (my mum says nosey; I do prefer curious – hell, as a journalist I think I can justify it as 'professionally curious').

One dull, grey Monday morning I got to my desk clutching a cup of coffee and a chocolate croissant (surely the only way to get through the start of a week) to find an email already waiting from him. It was short, to the point and exactly the kind of thing that set my mind in a frenzy and my fingers tapping out a flurry of questions in return.

I have plans for this weekend. A big challenge. I'm going to introduce you to something new.

I was burning with curiosity. The nerves had started in earnest and I was soon working at it like a knot, trying to unravel what the challenge could be from the (admittedly scant) information he would give me. The annoying thing was, I knew that he had told me this early in the week because he wanted the anticipation and nerves to increase as we edged closer to the weekend. But knowing that didn't stop me reacting exactly as he expected. I couldn't help it. Annoying brain. On Monday the only thing he would concede to my mostly-ignored questions was that:

It won't hurt in the way you're thinking. But I can't say it won't hurt at all.

I'll be honest, after the ginger incident I wasn't taking anything for granted. We'd already ascertained he could do things to me that I'd never even thought of. My curiosity drove me to distraction.

I tried to question him when his guard was down. Faux casually before he went to sleep. While we were eating dinner. Even while we were having sex. But he was having none of it. He just grinned at me, and got the kind of glint in his eye that made me feel excited and nervous in equal measure.

Even when the weekend finally arrived he made me wait. I spent all of Friday night half expecting him to jump me, or tell me to fetch something from the blanket box, which had become our de facto home for toys. But nothing. Saturday we spent most of the day playing computer games together on our laptops, and by Sunday I was half-convinced he'd forgotten, or changed his mind, or whatever he was planning was dependent on something he'd ordered and which hadn't arrived yet.

Silly Sophie.

We were sitting on the sofa watching nothing in particular on TV when he took my hand and stood up. He didn't look at me or say anything, but his meaning was clear. I followed him into the bedroom.

As he moved to the blanket box – *I knew it!* (knew what? I have no idea, but it was a vindication of sorts) – he spoke to me over his shoulder.

'Take your clothes off. All of them.'

His tone was brusque but, for now at least, any nerves were pushed aside by a sense of anticipation. I took my clothes off quickly, trying to peer past his back to see what he was removing from his box of tricks.

Once I was naked he turned to me, holding a couple of lengths of rope. He pushed me onto the bed and tied my wrists together and then tied them to the headboard. He then spread my legs open and tied each ankle to a corner of the bed, leaving me spread wide open.

Before Adam, I was relatively unused to being tied up. My exes had often used cuffs and on the rare occasions they did use rope it was in a perfunctory fashion. Adam was a rope aficionado. He loved shibari, and his ties were often elaborate, meticulous, with him occasionally loosening something that didn't sit right to then pull it back in place perfectly. He became completely focused on the job at hand when he tied me up and I loved to watch the look of concentration on his face. But even on that basis he was more disconnected from me now than usual. He moved my arms and legs as he wanted to, but his movements were businesslike, I was another plaything. It was an oddly hot thought. I suppose I should be grateful he didn't keep *me* in the blanket box.

He left the room briefly, and returned trailing wires. I was confused and a little nervous – my first thought was, 'Does whatever that is plug in at the mains?' Then he moved closer, lifting his arms to show me what he'd got.

Everyone's seen those machines. They're the kind of things they advertise on late-night TV aimed at people desperate to get fit but lacking the time or motivation to get to the gym. I've read the hyperbole, seen the Sunday supplement brochures, but always been a bit suspicious if I'm honest. Frankly, I have lard-arse tendencies brought about by a lifetime's love of cheese. I don't see how four sticky pads attached to my stomach are going to be able to work any 'muscles' hiding under the legacy of Cheddar.

When I'd first seen the TENS machine amid his stuff when we were unpacking I'd mocked Adam a little, but he told me it was good for treating muscle pain he got as a result of a recurring rugby injury. I was suddenly aware he had potentially left out a secondary use that might have been of interest to me. Git.

He placed a small circular pad on my breast, just beside my nipple. It was cold and sticky and I shivered slightly as he adjusted it. Then he added a second one to the other side of my already-erect nipple (let's say it was part nerves, part arousal). He moved to the other breast and did the same.

I was wary as he leaned down towards me, his breath tickling against my ear.

'Do you remember your safe word?'

My throat was dry and I wasn't sure I trusted myself to speak, so I nodded.

'Say it out loud.' I hesitated. He took my silence for stubbornness. 'Come on, there's no shame in saying it. Say it for me.' My jaw was clenched, and my nerves increased in the way they always did when he performed this almost ritualistic check. The word I had chosen – courtesy of an in-joke from a comedy show – was deliberately unalluring and faintly ridiculous. But it wasn't that I was worried about killing the moment or whatever, it was that this check inevitably pinpointed that whatever was about to happen was going to be a serious challenge for me. After a week of wondering about what he had in mind, all my wild theories had been blown out of the water with his first move. I couldn't second-guess him and had no idea what was coming next. This was a real step into the unknown, where I had to trust him and let him be my guide. I mentally cursed him for making the build-up even worse, then took a steadying breath, trying to calm myself down.

Then, through gritted teeth: 'Flugelhorn.' I told you it was unalluring.

Half a second after I'd spoken, I cried out loud. I couldn't help it. A sudden sharp pain ran across my nipples. I had a split second to think, 'He was right, this isn't a conventional pain, it feels different,' and then it hit me again. I don't cry out a lot – I'm usually a whimperer, and even then a grudging one, but every burst of pain that flashed across my skin wrenched a loud cry from my throat.

Fuck.

In the kind of random thought that flashes through my mind in these kinds of moments I suddenly thought, '*He uses this to feel better?*'

Over the next minute or so the pain came and went every few seconds. The relentless pulse made my nipples prickle and the soft flesh of my breasts sting.

He moved closer, and I glared at him, standing there with his little white plastic box, the black and red wires attached to my body. I noticed as well that there were a worrying number of knobs and buttons on the box. I could see where this was going.

He definitely wanted to play. He twisted a dial and suddenly my back was arching with the increased intensity and length of the pulse. Fuck. I let out a noise that can only be described as a mournful wail. He changed the programme, possibly to minimise any disruption to our neighbours.

After a moment of blessed relief, the pain began to build again. It started as a minor prickle, but as the seconds lengthened I began to bite my lip to try and stop the cry forming in my throat.

Adam watched me struggle against the rope, and grinned at me – the same kind of look he'd had when I gave him the remote-controlled egg. I had a flash of what he'd have looked like as a kid when he was given a Scalextric or some such. Hell, he was still a gadget fiend now, it's just his favourite toys included semi-naked women.

His fingers moved again on the box and I steeled myself for what was coming next. It was as though he wanted to see what reactions and noises he could elicit from me – what was hardest for me to handle.

More quickly than I expected he switched the machine off, pulling the sticky pads off my breasts and giving my nipples a quick kiss as he did so.

His smile was getting wider with every passing minute and it made me feel an odd mix of affection at how much fun he was having and nerves at what exactly he was up to. I was right to be suspicious.

'Right. Let's get started shall we?'

What? I thought we were finished. Shit.

He placed the four pads in two sets of two at the very top of my inner thigh, tantalisingly (and, admittedly, a little worryingly) close to my cunt. Control box in hand, he sat himself down on the bed next to my prone body. He had the look in his eyes that simultaneously makes me wet and nervous. His thumb flicked a couple of switches and then the movement started.

The initial shock (if you'll forgive the pun) of the feeling tickling my thighs made me jump, even though I'd just felt the same sensations in my breasts. I squirmed a little in the rope, and got a smirk. But then I had time to adjust to the sensation.

At the lowest setting the tingling felt not dissimilar to

my rabbit vibrator being run along my inner thigh. It was pleasant, tickling, soothing almost. I even began to relax into it, enjoying being teased within my bonds.

I don't know how long we lay there that way, but I was blissed out by the time the sensation changed. The strength of the vibration increased – a quick look at Adam's smile made me realise I wasn't imagining it – and suddenly it didn't feel like a vibrator running across my skin, but as if my skin itself was properly vibrating – which of course it was as the current ran through it. The feeling wasn't unpleasant, but was certainly a step up from before. I started to move more in the ropes in spite of my attempts to stay still, squirming against the sensation.

The next half an hour or so was ridiculously intense. I had seriously underestimated that little machine. It had more pulsing patterns than the highest-spec rabbit I'd ever owned (and that one had thirty-one speeds – I'm a gadget geek, I can't help it). Some of the patterns were teasing, taking me almost there; some were full-on, leaving me writhing and whimpering a little to myself, although if you'd asked me I'd have been hard pressed to tell you if it was in pleasure or pain. And then of course there was the power dial. Initially we were using the different pulse pattern programmes at lower intensity – as, frankly, you should when you're trying anything new and feeling a little nervous. However, by the time a sheen of sweat had started forming between my shoulder blades and my thighs were damp with proof that, actually, any nerves I did have about trying this had dissipated, Adam was happy to ramp things up a little higher.

It was a surprisingly innocuous setting, used at evilly high levels, that was the most painful and shocking. Adam nearly had to prise me off the ceiling afterwards. One burst on and then a few moments' respite. You'd think it would be easy to withstand, one quick burst and then relief. Yes? No. At higher levels the feeling of the electricity running through my body felt like tiny needle pin pricks. The feeling was a different kind of pain to the catharsis of a caning or a good session with the belt, and afterwards the memory of it faded quickly, but in that moment as it assaulted my thighs and the edge of my cunt it felt excruciating, like the most difficult thing I had ever experienced. The moments of rest just made my heart beat faster and my hands tremble more, as I knew the relief would be punctured quickly and my cries would start again. If he'd been torturing me for information, he would have got everything he needed and more. He told me afterwards – with a kind of smug pride – that he had seen my fingers clench into fists and my toes curl as I processed the pain. It didn't surprise me.

Thankfully he wasn't a sadist at heart, so eventually he tired of watching my lip wobble as I tried to work through the pain, my inner monologue urging me on, telling me that I need only last a few more seconds until it stopped. And then started again. By the time he'd finished with me, my mouth was dry and my throat was a little hoarse. And I hadn't even had an orgasm yet.

The orgasm was an interesting one (as I suppose all orgasms are). I'd always assumed electrosex was a form of D/s edgeplay, and certainly in the right context and with the right person at the controls it gives the opportunity to inflict sensation so intense it can be painful yet not leave any marks, in a way that Jack Bauer himself would be proud of. That said, at the lower levels the sensation is much more about pleasure – in fact if we're talking about 'edgeplay' as a concept then that moment where the pleasure becomes so intense as to be painful can be hugely fun to play with. After a lot of fiddling, Adam found the optimum setting to push my buttons. It was an intense, regular pulsing that increased in strength, and was set at a level that meant that when it reached the strongest part of the cycle there was a couple of seconds of agonising pain before the soothing bliss of the lower levels returned. My inner masochist was in heaven, while the constant shifts in sensation meant I was squirming against the bed in a desperate way, which made him happy too.

I don't think I'd have come from the sensation of the TENS pads alone, at least not placed where they were. While the focal point of the electricity zinging through me was close to my cunt, it wasn't intense or focused enough to bring me off. But when Adam slipped a glass dildo embarrassingly easily inside me and then leaned round to play with my clit while he fucked me with it, it took just a few seconds to push me over the edge, and when I fell it was loud, long and intense. I like to think I'm comfortable with my own body and know how to bring myself off, but even on my best day, at my horniest, and with the best my toy drawer has to offer, I've not ever felt an orgasm quite like that. The leg-wobbling aftermath continued as he pulled out the dildo, wiped his sticky fingers on my arse, unstuck the pads, and then began the arduous task of undoing all the rope securing my arms and legs. For a long while afterwards I was a ball of nerve endings, incapable of moving, although eventually I did because, frankly, after all that it felt a bit rude not to thank Adam somehow.

We lay cuddled together for long enough that my breathing had returned to normal, his hands stroking my back almost hypnotically. Finally, I crawled down his body and took him in my mouth – an obvious but fairly effective way of saying thank you for something so fiendish and so fun. If the size of his erection was anything to go by, I wasn't the only one who had enjoyed it, a thought that made me smile as I urged him deeper into my mouth, running my tongue along him and enjoying the sense of regaining a little control of things.

I took my time, enjoying the feeling of him in my mouth, loving his reactions and feeling like he deserved a little spoiling of his own (although my form of spoiling didn't have the frisson of delicious meanness that his did).

'Oh, Sophie,' he whispered as he tangled his hands in my hair, holding me still as he came. My heart swelled, and my ego felt a little smug. I figured it was OK because Adam was smug 85 per cent of the time when we did anything sexual (and that's being conservative). Hell, maybe it was catching.

I crawled back up the bed and tucked myself into the curve of his arm. He kissed the top of my head.

'You OK?'

I smiled. These quiet moments were something I had come to love – they were a sign of Adam's concern for me, and also functioned, in the nicest possible way, as a kind of post-coital post-mortem where he learned about the things I enjoyed the most, and the things I found most difficult to cope with. He was always loving and kind, even at his meanest, but no more so than in these moments when we talked frankly and happily about what had happened.

Of course, when we'd just done something filthy I could barely look at him without blushing, so a lot of the time I was whispering my responses into his chest.

'I'm great thank you. That was amazing. Really intense.'

'Not too much?'

'No, just right. Bearable. Well, not bearable. At points it was unbearable.' I broke off and sighed as I tried to pull together my thoughts, which is difficult at the best of times but even more so when I'm returning from my submissive headspace. It's like part of my brain is still trying to process how I feel about what happened, so explaining it to anyone else is like trying to nail custard to the wall. 'It's a weird one. I want to be pushed to the point where I don't think I can take any more, and then pushed a little bit further to prove that I can, even though I think I can't. You do that. You know what I can take.'

He chuckled. 'I think I'm beginning to know that, yes.' He kissed me again. 'You were so brave. I love it when you're all stoic and trying to withstand the pain. Also, watching you struggle when I've got you tied up? That's not getting old.'

I laughed in mock surprise. 'Really? You surprise me. I do have one question, though.'

His voice was curious. 'Go on.'

I felt a bit sheepish saying it, which is odd. 'What do you think it would have felt like if you'd fucked me while the electricity was pulsing through me?'

He leaned up to look down at me. 'You're amazing. Whenever I think of something filthy to do you've always got some idea to make it more twisted. It's brilliant.'

I smiled at him. 'I could say the same about you. It does make for some interesting times.'

'That it does, gorgeous, that it does.' He pulled the duvet up round my shoulders. 'We shall clearly have to experiment to see what it feels like to fuck that way.'

As I drifted off to sleep, I marvelled at what I'd found with Adam. I know it probably sounds daft, but I had never really anticipated having a boyfriend who I could live with, love, do all the usual day-to-day stuff with, and who would then fuck me fifteen ways to Sunday. I felt so incredibly lucky.

When I went for drinks with Tom one night after work a few weeks later I was still full of the joys of the honeymoon period. After a pretty shitty few months in the aftermath of my break-up with James, I was happier than I had ever been. Knowing Tom and Charlotte were having similar amounts of fun just made me feel even more lucky – not only had I found a partner who was evil and lovely in equal measure, but their relationship seemed to be going from strength to strength too.

Or so I thought. It turned out Thomas wasn't fibbing when he'd texted that things weren't always as they seemed.

The evening started fairly well. We ordered the first of a few beers, found a booth and settled down for a bit of a catch-up. He was telling me about the latest developments at work and a promotion he was in the process of applying for. He asked after my mum and I told him how her recovery from her knee operation was progressing. We argued a bit about TV shows we were both watching. It was as easy-going and full of banter as it had always been, and I felt a surge of affection for my friend – I promise it wasn't the beer talking.

'I'm so glad we've had time to catch up. It feels like it's been ages,' I said. 'It's lovely that I've got Adam and you've got Charlotte, and us all doing stuff together is surprisingly comfortable all things considered, but it's been a while since we've gone out just the two of us.'

Tom nodded. 'Probably not since the aftermath of your break-up with James. It's funny, I've never stayed friends with a girl after we've stopped sleeping together.' He raised his glass in mock toast. 'To ex-friends with benefits.'

I clinked my glass but shook my head. 'We're not ex-friends. We have ex-benefits. It's not the same thing.'

Tom grinned at me. 'Pedant. That's the kind of smart-mouthed comment that I'd have caned you for back in the day.'

I stuck my tongue out at him. 'Well, those days are most definitely gone. I don't think either Adam or Charlotte would be especially impressed.'

He smiled. 'I know Adam wouldn't be, but I'm not sure Charlotte would mind.'

I stayed silent. One thing a life in journalism has taught

me is if you don't know what to say, letting a silence run will usually encourage someone else to fill it. Tom didn't disappoint.

'We have an open relationship, you know.'

I took a sip of my beer. 'Oh really?' I'd kind of guessed they were open to having fun with other people, mostly from passing comments Charlotte had made about play parties and club nights they'd been to, but I didn't know the details. I wasn't really sure it was my business any more.

Tom clearly wanted to talk, though. 'Charlotte's amazing. Sexy, funny, good-hearted. She's a great girl. In the last year we've done so much stuff that previously I'd wanted to do but never had the chance to. Threesomes.' At this point I blushed, remembering my experiences with the two of them, way back at the beginning of their relationship. 'Public play, heavy pain, 24/7 stuff. I've taken her to parties and made her fuck other guys in front of me. She's dominated other women, not just you.' I rolled my eyes. 'It's incredible. She's incredible. She's fulfilled almost all my fantasies.'

He tailed off. I wasn't sure what he was getting at, but he wasn't saying anything more. I cleared my throat.

'Surely "almost all" your fantasies is pretty good? And as boundaries change you're going to probably end up doing more, if that's what you both want. After all –'

'That's not what I mean, Soph.'

I was confused. Tom isn't great at talking about his feelings at the best of times. Having this kind of emotional conversation at all was as surreal as talking to a sea lion. At this point it made about the same amount of sense. 'Well, what *do* you mean?'

'I love her. I'm in love with her. And she likes me. She likes me *a lot*.' His face screwed up and he used his fingers to make stabbing quotes marks in the air. 'But we aren't a couple, not really. She doesn't want to be one.'

He looked disconsolate. I put my hand across the table and squeezed his. I honestly didn't know what to say. 'But I thought you were effectively dating now?'

He shook his head.

'We see each other most weekends. We have a lot of fun. We meet up with you guys together. We go to all these kink events. But we don't really talk about much emotional stuff. It's mostly sex. And she's seeing other people.'

I leaned forward in my chair. 'Are you sure she's seeing other people? How do you know?'

His smile was pained. 'She's told me. To be fair to her, she's told me she's OK with me doing the same. She just wants to have fun.'

I cast about for some kind of way to clarify. 'Is she poly? Is that what she means? Does she want to be in relationships with several people?'

He shook his head. 'If it were that, I'd give it some serious thought if we could all make it work. It's not polyamory. She just doesn't want a serious relationship at the moment.'

Tom looked so downhearted it made me feel sad for him. He never really talked much about his feelings – I'd certainly never seen him wear his heart on his sleeve to this extent.

'She's pretty much limitless, Soph. She is so filthy, so sexy. She'll fulfil all my fantasies. She'll literally do pretty much anything I tell her to do. But I can't order her to love me. And she doesn't.'

We finished our drinks in a sombre mood. All my attempts to reassure him about Charlotte were scuppered by one fundamental truth – that he was right, he could dominate her to fulfil his every physical whim, but he couldn't change how she felt emotionally. Poor Tom.

Chapter Eleven

As the months passed – and we finally unpacked all our belongings – our life together began to take on a rhythm. It was straightforward, no-fuss, and had a soothing ebb and flow to it. I tended to cook of an evening because I usually got in from work first, but Adam would stack the dishwasher and then spend hours at the weekend marinating things and cooking elaborate and delicious meals, although he'd always make sure the kitchen was free if I had the urge to bake. Meanwhile he did the cleaning, I did the organising, ensuring his godchildren got their birthday presents and his grandparents' wedding anniversary was marked, and everything pootled along nicely. It might feel ironic when, in sexual terms, there was such a strong D/s element – and thus an inherent power imbalance – to our love life, but in every other way we were equals. We were loving, happy, cheering each other's highs and supporting each other through the lows.

It was just unfortunate when suddenly Adam's career stumbled slightly.

He'd been working in a copywriting agency for eight years, and had been promoted several times, when suddenly they were bought up by a larger agency. As Adam was in a managerial role that was duplicated by a worker from the larger company he knew as soon as the merger was announced that his role might be at risk. It's safe to say that neither of us expected things to move so quickly, though.

I got home from work one night to find him already sat at the kitchen table with a mug of tea. I put my grocery bags on the side and leaned over to kiss him hello, and he leaned into me, his arms enveloping me in a hug. I wrapped my arms round him for a couple of seconds, before kissing the top of his head and arching away to look at him.

'Are you OK? What's up?'

He pressed a kiss to my breast and sighed softly. 'They made me an offer today.'

I was, admittedly, a bit dazed and confused. As I said, we really weren't expecting this straight away. 'Who did?'

'The MD. They've made me an offer for voluntary redundancy.'

I hugged him again, pulling him close, my mind whirring. 'Really? Seriously? Fuck. Are you OK?' I know, it's a stupid question, but that's the kind of inane thing your brain flings up when something like this happens. Trust me, I too wish I'd said something more profound.

He nodded. 'I'm fine. But we need to have a think about what happens now.'

The offer was, on paper, a tempting one. Adam had talked often about his frustration with the management structure, even about setting up on his own. They were willing to pay him six months' salary to go immediately, he wouldn't even have to work more than minimal notice. As redundancy settlements are tax free they would effectively give him eight or nine months' money up front to go. If he got a new job, or even started freelancing and building customers for his own agency before he worked through that money, then he was in a good place. I knew what I'd do if it were me, but I also knew that, while I loved him and would support him in whatever he wanted to do, it had to be his choice.

Thankfully, he could see that taking redundancy made the most sense, and went in the next day to negotiate terms (he even ended up with a little bit more; I was very proud). But as he pointed out darkly when we toasted his new beginning less than a week later, it was somewhat ironic that in the time we had been seeing each other there had been two batches of redundancies at my paper – sadly not an industry rarity – and I had made it through both unscathed, while he ended up the one with the pay-off. All in all, though, he seemed to be dealing with it fine. He was positive about the opportunities the move offered, and undoubtedly the cushion of money sitting in his current account helped with any pangs of anxiety.

Things changed a little, though, in the first few weeks after he finished at his old company. He'd applied for a few jobs, arranged meetings with ex-colleagues and other agencies, so he was out and about at various points. But when he was home he was amazing: I came home to epic dinners most nights, the washing was up-to-date, and even a few DIY jobs around the house got done now he had time on his hands. It was brilliant. He wanted to keep busy, was laid-back about how long it was likely to take to organise a new role and wanted to make the most of the weeks he was free. Who was I to argue?

He also plotted a lot of rude fun. He bought toys

online, happy in the knowledge that there'd be no need for a trip to the dreaded sorting office because he would be around to sign for his latest goodies. He would send me emails at work hinting at what he'd bought, telling what to expect when I got home. Or I would get home and find him lurking with a twinkle in his eye and a plan in mind. It ranged from the abrupt and violent – grabbing me as I walked through the door for kisses and under-coat groping – to the gentle and loving – one grey, wintery day I got in, drenched through, to find a warm bath already run and Adam keen to help me out of my wet clothes and pass me a glass of wine. Definitely not a hardship.

Even with my horizons continually expanding thanks to my lovely dominant boyfriend, there were still things that left me somewhat perplexed when he first introduced them. That was how I found myself loitering outside a pet shop in an out-of-town shopping centre on a drizzly Saturday morning.

It was cold. We'd had our usual weekend lie-in – well, it was a sort-of lie-in: we were both distressingly incapable of sleeping in beyond 8 a.m. even when we didn't have to worry about the alarm going off. After a leisurely fuck, not especially D/s-ish but still lovely, he'd got up and flung a pair of jeans at me.

'Come on. Let's go shopping.'

I was confused. Partly because we were in our own little age of austerity, trying to ensure no unnecessary dipping into his redundancy money, and partly because I knew we had plenty of food in for the weekend. As he chucked a jumper at me I stuck my tongue out at him.

'Choosing what I wear? How überdomly of you.' He pulled the covers away and I stood up, grumbling to myself. He kissed me on the nose.

'Now now, don't be bratty. Just for that, I think you should put your jeans on without knickers.'

I looked at him for long moments, trying to figure out if this was sarcastic Adam or gearing-up-to-some-kind-of-rudeness Adam. Then the penny dropped. It was both.

I mock sighed, although we both knew that my pulse had started racing a little at the undercurrent of this supposedly innocent shopping trip.

'Fine.' I started shimmying into my jeans. As I did them up, he put his arms round me and pulled me into a deep kiss. He was smiling when we broke apart.

'Good girl.'

I felt myself grin back at him in spite of myself. Damn it. I picked up a bra and walked over to the jumper on the bed. He was up to something. I knew it.

When we pulled into the car park of the pet superstore I looked over at him with raised eyebrows. He pretended not to see and got out of the car. I followed, already suspicious about where this was going. We don't own any pets, not even a goldfish, so, unless he was about to buy me a puppy, I knew why we were here. He'd mentioned it before; it was one of the rude things we whispered about as we lay in bed at night, turning each other on with rude fantasies and ideas. It wasn't breaking any limits, and it was something I was intrigued by – though I was also quite embarrassed at the prospect of wandering into

Pets at Home on a Saturday morning in order to fulfil a fantasy.

As we walked up the stairs to the automatic door I couldn't stop myself asking the question, half under my breath. 'Why do we have to buy this stuff here? All the other new bits you're buying you've been getting online.'

He heard me and turned round with the kind of smile that made me tempted to push him back down the steps. 'Now, where's the fun in that? I wanted you with me.'

Git.

I glared at him, and he took my hand. His fingers were stroking my palm, although I wasn't sure if it was to try and assuage the nerves he knew underpinned my fury, or to stop me bolting back to the car or hiding in the craft warehouse over the way. Maybe now was the time for me to take up cross stitch.

Of course, I knew the worst thing would be to look nervous and guilty. We were only in a pet shop. It wasn't a Soho sex shop for goodness' sake (and even some of those are looking rather classy nowadays). I looked at my shoes as much as possible, almost taking out a display of bird feeders as I did so. He led me to the back of the shop.

We stood in front of a wall with cages displayed on it. They ranged from something small enough for a rabbit right up to something big enough for a Great Dane. Or a Sophie. I remembered the cage in the kink cottage and blushed. Adam leaned in behind me to get a closer look at the dimensions and price ticket of the cage that was holding my attention.

'One day we'll have a house big enough to store one of these, so I can put you inside it whenever I want to.'

I blushed at his words. I didn't say anything, but I felt the twitch between my legs that showed I wasn't averse to the idea. I wasn't going to give him the satisfaction of knowing it, though. I muttered noncommittally and walked further along the aisle. He followed but stopped me again to look at something else.

'Of course we'd need a big cushion to go in the bottom of it.'

There was a couple with a Yorkshire terrier on a lead stood a little way down, certainly near enough to overhear any response. I decided discretion was the better form of valour. I humoured him.

'Obviously.'

He was looking mischievous and was clearly having fun. I felt my lips quirk in spite of myself. Two could play at that game. I aimed for casual, studied indifference, and wandered over to look at some adorable long-eared rabbits. My calm lasted approximately four seconds, long enough for him to lead me over to the pet bowls.

'Pick one.'

I stared at them. Through them. Around them. They all looked like pet bowls. Some of them were ridiculously priced. One of them had PRINCESS written on it in a kind of diamante. People bought those for their pets? My mind was drifting a little when his voice interrupted my thoughts.

'Come on. We can't leave until we get a bowl.'

We could leave then? Fine. I snatched the nearest non-diamante, reasonably priced bowl I could find, a simple white china thing, and thrust it into his hands.

'Also a collar and lead.'

What. A. Cock.

He led me over to the collars and leads. It'd been a long time since I'd had a family dog, and when we were getting accessories for Barry there certainly wasn't this array. Leather, suede, patterned, plain, studded. More bloody diamantes. In spite of myself, I began studying them, curious as to which felt most right for me, and then began to feel a little concerned that *any* of them felt right for me. Pet play had been my idea in the first place, born mostly of how safe, simple and unexpectedly erotic it had felt in the confines in the cage. I hadn't quite expected this, though.

Almost without me realising it, my fingers had moved towards a thick collar made of brown suede. I stroked it, and suddenly Adam's voice was right behind me, his tone low.

'Do you like that one?'

My voice was hesitant. 'I just thought it looked soft and nice somehow.'

He unhooked it from the display and I dropped my hand down awkwardly.

'It's really long. Are you sure it'll fit?'

I glared at him in spite of my embarrassment. 'I don't think it's something you can try on,' I hissed.

He waggled his eyebrows and stuck his tongue out at me but thankfully moved down the aisle to find the matching lead. It was simple brown leather with a plaited part where the looped handle was. I remember thinking I liked it, and then giving myself a mental shake for caring.

Having picked all three things, we could finally leave.

As we approached the till I thrust everything into his hands – if he was making me do this he could definitely pay for it. I know we could have been buying it for an actual pet, but previous experiences had taught me I had nothing like a poker face. I knew my expression would give me away if I approached the counter, so I lurked, pretending to read a display about a spray that encouraged good behaviour in dogs. I wondered if it worked on boyfriends.

Meanwhile, I could hear Adam making small talk with the cute girl serving him. He easily made up a story about our imaginary Alsatian and made her laugh – apparently his dog didn't always follow instructions but was mostly a good pet. I wanted to take a run up to kick him in his backside – making fun of me while flirting with another woman. He was lucky I didn't bite his leg.

He picked up the bag from the counter and looked round to see where I was. I walked towards the door and he joined me, taking my hand and leading me outside. I called him an arse and he laughed out loud, leaning over and kissing me on the forehead. I melted a bit, which made me angry with myself as much as him.

Once we'd got home he laid the collar, lead and bowl out on the coffee table, displaying them for me. He then walked out of the room, telling me to stay. It took a split second for me to get the double meaning, by which time my folded arms and unimpressed facial expression were somewhat academic as he'd disappeared from sight. He returned a few minutes later with a pile of cushions, pillows and blankets.

He carefully laid everything out on the floor in front of the sofa and I realised he was making a little bed – no prizes for guessing who for. I suppose I should have thanked my lucky stars he hadn't bought one of those big cushions after all.

He sank down on the sofa.

'Strip.' His tone was businesslike. Almost dismissive.

I'd been naked in front of him a thousand times by now, easily. He'd seen me naked just a couple of hours ago. Hell, he shared a bed with me naked every night, barring extreme wintry weather worthy of fleecy pyjamas. But when he stared at me intently like this I always felt uncomfortable. I took my jumper and bra off and then fumbled with the buttons on my jeans. Finally I pulled them down, trying to ignore the flush of embarrassment – and his matching smirk – as I bared myself to him. I tried not to shift from foot to foot, which was a sure-fire way of betraying my nerves.

'Get down on your knees and crawl over here.'

It took a few seconds before I could actually move. The idea of doing something so humiliating was hot in the abstract, but when faced with the prospect of actually doing it, my first instinct was to baulk, to prevaricate, to suggest doing it another time. Make some tea. Do that bit of freelance reviewing I'd been putting off. Anything else.

He sat patiently, watching me. He didn't say anything else, which just made me more cross. He knew he didn't *need* to say anything. He knew I would do it, even while I wasn't sure. Arrogant arse. I sighed and gingerly sank to the floor. I saw Adam nod in approval as I began to move slowly across the carpet until I was kneeling on the floor by his feet.

I kept my head down, not ready to look at him. Unfortunately he knew this trick, so when I reached him he stroked all my hair out of my face, holding it in a makeshift ponytail and pulling it slightly so I had to make eye contact. I blushed, feeling small.

'Hold your hair for me.'

I did so. He undid my necklace – a birthday gift from him, and the only piece of jewellery I wore – and slipped it into his pocket. We looked at each other for long moments, and then slowly his fingers moved to my throat and he buckled the collar tightly round my neck. The feeling of the suede at my throat gave me goosebumps.

Collars are funny things. Obviously they're a mainstay of the BDSM cliché but they weren't something I was ever inclined to try. My submission – whoever I give it to – is a private thing. I don't need to wear a collar to show the world. In lots of ways the necklace Adam gave me, while subtle enough to wear under my work clothes, was a sign of his love and, yes, his dominance. I wore it all the time; my throat felt naked without it. But to anyone other than us it was just a necklace. I was more than happy with that. Usually.

The suede of the collar was about two inches wide and made it feel difficult to move my neck up and down as readily as usual. It felt constricting. Heavy. Soft. Lovely. Challenging. I swallowed, or tried to, and the collar felt even tighter. I sat, staring at the floor, just breathing in and out, getting used to it. Or trying to.

Adam leaned forward and attached the lead with

a 'click' that felt so loud it made me flinch. He took a handful of my hair and we began the dialogue we always have before our most challenging play.

'Do you remember your safe word?'

I nodded. He smiled.

'Good. Apart from that one word I don't want you saying anything else. Understand?'

I nodded again. Being silent wouldn't really be a problem for me. I usually found it harder to speak when he was humiliating me.

He stood up and started to walk away from the sofa, pulling me along by the lead. He took me for a walk all around the flat, tugging from time to time to make sure I kept to his pace – at times he was moving so fast that I had to shuffle quite quickly to keep up.

Eventually he led me back to the sofa and told me to get onto my bed. If I'd been allowed to speak I'd probably have made some smart comment at that, but as I wasn't, I crawled onto the surprisingly comfy pile of cushions, curling up so that I would fit. He lay down on the sofa and we started to watch some television.

After a few minutes he absent-mindedly reached down and started to stroke my hair. He ran his fingers along my cheek, and then scratched his fingernail along behind my ear. My ears and the nape of my neck are two of the erogenous zones that would make me purr. It took all my effort not to make a noise as his fingers meandered between them, but I lay there, enjoying his touch, my mind drifting. It was peaceful, calming, and eventually even the collar round my neck didn't feel such a big deal.

I don't know how long we stayed in companionable

silence before he stood up and walked out of the room, picking the bowl up from the coffee table as he passed it. My heart started beating faster, my nerves rising. This was the moment I was worried I wouldn't be able to cope with, the humiliation going too far in spite of the eroticism and odd intimacy.

Adam came back with a drink for himself and a bowl of water for me. He was also carrying a packet of small biscuits.

He put the bowl down in front of me and told me to drink, but he didn't stand over me waiting to see if I would do it. Instead he settled back on his sofa, sipping from his Coke and crunching a biscuit. His hand didn't return to stroke me, though. I felt oddly bereft at the loss, missing his touch.

I lay, still and frozen, staring at the bowl which, thanks to the angle at which he had placed it, pretty much filled my field of vision.

Once he had finished his drink and placed his empty glass on the table, he looked down at me. I hadn't moved. I couldn't move. I'm guessing he knew I wouldn't.

He sat up, feet on the floor, and leaned down to look me in the eye.

'Are you going to use your safe word?'

Mindful of his warning to stay quiet, and not inclined to get myself into any more trouble, I silently shook my head.

'Then do as you're told and drink.' A pause. 'Or don't. It's OK. We have all day. Eventually you'll get thirsty enough that you'll have to.'

His voice wasn't harsh. If anything, his tone was oddly

soothing, but his words were matter-of-fact. He knew this was hard for me but was determined to make me do it. In a way, that made it easier. He wanted this, he wanted me to do this. If I couldn't be brave enough to try this for myself, I would do it for him, to please him.

So I did.

I lowered my head and my lips touched the cool water. I was glad my hair fell in front of my face to hide me but I realised too late that it was getting wet as I took a slightly slurpy-sounding sip. He reached down and pulled my hair back into the ponytail again. I noticed he had my lead on his wrist once more.

I took a couple more sips from the bowl, in the hope it would get easier. I managed to dip my face in the water – so, no, not getting less embarrassing. I looked up at him, my gaze pleading. He smiled at me and sat back on the sofa. He pulled me by the lead, away from the bowl, so that I was sat between his legs.

He began stroking my hair again and the movement soothed me. 'Good pet.' I stiffened for a moment, but he said nothing more, and slowly I began to relax, resting my head on his knee, basking in his attention and praise.

A while later he reached for the biscuits. I eyed him warily.

He put one in his palm and held his hand out in front of me. Instinctively I moved my head down and picked it up with my mouth. Only as I bit into it did I have a mental jolt. My hands were free. I could have reached for it – even if he'd told me off, there had been nothing to stop me from trying. But instinctively, I had used my mouth. I couldn't decide if this was a good or a bad thing. Then he called me a good pet again and I decided the best thing was not to think at all. The simplicity and the quiet companionship of what we were doing felt lovely, but there was a prickle of embarrassment with it, a kind of humiliation I couldn't shake. I wasn't sure if I loved this or hated it, but I noticed a bulge in Adam's trousers, so I think it was fair to say I could guess how he felt about the whole thing.

He caught me looking and smiled, asking me if I wanted his cock. I nodded without daring to look at him and he unfastened the buttons on his jeans, pulling himself out. He gave the lead a little tug but I didn't need the invitation, I moved forward and opened my mouth to take him in. But he stopped me.

'Not like that. You need to lick it.'

I blushed. Don't get me wrong, my blow-job repertoire involved a fair amount of licking. But not like this. Never like this. Still, who was I to argue? Not that I could, anyway, what with the whole not-talking thing. Fine.

I blushed as I ran my tongue up and down his shaft, swirling around the top to get his pre-cum. I lapped just below the head of his cock, making him stiffen and gasp. Then I moved lower, licking his balls, loving the sound of him moaning.

I figured eventually he would put his cock in my mouth and I was sure he wasn't too far from orgasm, but after a long time he stopped me and told me to turn round. I did and he made me crawl a few paces away from him while he kept hold of the lead.

He got on his knees behind me and placed the tip of his cock between my legs, almost inside me but just not quite. It was torture feeling him there for such a long time but I did my best not to move until he told me to push backwards, pulling on my lead as he did so. I sank myself back onto his cock and groaned – the first noise I'd made in ages.

The noise he made in response can only be described as a growl of pleasure. 'God, Sophie, you're so fucking wet.'

He wasn't wrong.

He chuckled. 'I love that you're loving this.'

I stared at the ground, knowing he was right, but wanting to lower my head, just to give myself a moment to process it without him seeing. But I knew he saw everything; sometimes he saw too much.

He pulled on the lead, dragging me back to him. He didn't move his hips, though.

'Fuck me. Show me how much you're enjoying this.'

I smiled. This I could do, collar and lead or not. I moved my hips forward before sliding back down his shaft. He seemed to want me to take my time so that's what I did. For a long time I kept up a steady but very slow rhythm, moving forward until his cock almost escaped me and then pushing back down until his pelvis met my arse.

After all this time I knew his reactions well and could tell when he was fighting off his orgasm. He kept making me hold still so he could recover slightly, and I was an obedient pet and did so, although I made sure to move my hips just a little at those points – sometimes I think it's as good for him to fight for control as it is for me.

Of course, the fucking, on top of everything else, took its effect on me too, and soon I was fighting off my own orgasm. We both wanted it to last and, even though his knees must have ached as much as mine, we just kept slowly fucking each other.

It was him that broke first. Usually he loved being teased and could withstand it much longer than me (I think it's because he's usually more patient), but he just didn't seem able to hold back any longer and as I pushed back on him he thrusted forward, suddenly fucking me hard. Of course I echoed his tempo, and soon my orgasm was building momentum too.

I had a moment of sudden panic – if we were doing something particularly intense on the D/s front he tended to prefer me to ask permission for my orgasm, but how can you do that when you can't speak? Fortunately Adam knows me well, sometimes better than I know myself. Through deep breaths he told me I was allowed to come, which is just as well because seconds later we both cried out.

For a moment he stayed where he was, and then he leaned back on the sofa, putting his head back, catching his breath.

Unthinkingly, I crawled back to my bed and curled up once again.

I don't know how long I slept for but I must have been out within seconds of lying down. When I awoke he was in front of me again – though this time I noticed he'd taken a couple of my cushions to protect his knees. I smiled to myself; he clearly wasn't as used to kneeling as I was.

His cock was hard again and just inches from my face. His hand was between my legs. I could feel and hear how wet I was as he pushed his fingers inside me. As he did so, he began talking to me, telling me how dirty I was for getting turned on by being treated like an animal, and how I clearly made a good little whore pet. His words made my skin burn but I clenched around his fingers.

He pulled out and then pushed his fingers into my mouth, making me taste our mixed juices, a reminder of both our pleasure.

His hand moved back between my legs as he pushed his cock into my mouth. I tried to use my tongue on him but he wasn't interested in that. He was just going to use my mouth – fuck it while he roughly fingered me.

His thumb found my clit and applied pressure. Within seconds I came. He gave me a moment to begin to get my breath back but didn't take his cock out of my mouth. Soon he was back to fucking my face, his hand in my hair, choking me as he pushed into my throat. He stiffened and filled my mouth.

This time he didn't leave me on my makeshift bed but pulled me up onto the sofa with him. He took my lead off but as he tried to remove the collar, I placed my hand on his. I liked wearing it, and went back to sleep in his arms with it still around my neck.

The dynamic of pet play was an interesting one – it felt liberating, mostly because I wasn't expected to speak, which is a relief in the most embarrassing of scenarios he comes up with. It wasn't about pretending to be an animal specifically, obviously, but more about the simplicity of it. He had even more control than usual, and we both enjoyed that and it felt less jarring than our foray into 24/7 D/s had.

In a lot of ways, the closeness of our relationship, the D/s side and the ordinary boyfriend/girlfriend side, helped make the changes in Adam's work life easier to bear. If nothing else, stuff like this distracted him for a few hours.

Also, it was bloody fun.

Chapter Twelve

As the weeks passed and Adam's various interviews didn't result in any job offers, I began to see a slight change in him. Not much – fear not, this isn't going to turn into some made-for-TV-drama-style relationship – but suddenly there were moments of nerves. I caught him looking pensive. Worried. Sad.

We were actually pretty lucky really. I brought in a decent salary, certainly enough to cover the rent and bills – not least because I'd been used to paying those on my own before we moved in together. We could keep ticking along in the short term pretty well even if his money ran out, and thankfully we were a long way from that happening yet. It didn't stop him getting frustrated, though. It all started with a row over a takeaway pizza, of all things.

I'd got in late from work and Adam had been out at an interview so neither of us had sorted out anything for dinner. We arrived home pretty simultaneously, and he picked up the post and riffled through it while I shrugged out of my coat and went into the kitchen to open the fridge and begin pulling out the makings of a meal. He followed me in, half-reading a letter.

'Soph, don't bother cooking. Shall we order a takeaway? I fancy a pizza.'

I looked at the eggs, vegetables and herbs I'd put on the side, mentally weighing up whether it was worth dropping

£20 on the cost of a pizza and associated accoutrements (because if you're going the takeaway route, a pizza without garlic bread is a travesty).

I gestured at the chopping board I'd just put on the side. 'We don't need to. I can make a Spanish omelette in ten minutes or so. It'll be quicker than waiting for the pizza to arrive.'

He looked up at me from his letter, his eyes assessing me in the same way they did when he was trying to decide how I was going to react in a D/s scene.

'It's OK, I don't mind waiting. We could open a bottle of wine, wait in style.'

I turned to the knife block, picked out a vegetable knife and went back to the board. 'Nah, week-night pizza is a bit decadent. I don't mind cooking.'

He moved in behind me and gently took the knife and put it down, twirling me round to look at him. He kissed the bridge of my nose and smiled down at me. 'Soph, we can have a pizza. It won't break the bank.'

I looked at him. He knew me too well. This whole 'able to tell what I was thinking' thing was seriously hot (albeit also bloody annoying at times) in sexual situations. It made him, for the most part, a thoughtful and sensitive boyfriend. But on the rare occasions I did want to hide something it made it difficult. Times like now.

I sighed and put the knife away. I smiled at him, but it felt forced. I just hoped he couldn't tell. 'OK, let's get pizza.'

I grabbed my tablet and began looking up the menu online. He leaned in behind me and we began discussing the relative merits of barbecue sauce on the base (a must in my book) as we chose our meal. I put the order through and then went to grab my card to put in the details to pay.

'What are you doing?' he asked as I rummaged through my handbag.

'Ordering the pizza,' I said, my tone snappier than I meant it to be.

'You don't have to do that,' he said, his tone snappier than mine. 'I'll pay for the bloody thing. I suggested we have pizza, I'll get it.'

'You don't need to, I'm ordering it. I can pay.'

He grabbed the tablet from my hand. 'I'll pay for the pizza.'

I went to grab it back, aware this was a bit of an unseemly tussle, and that it wasn't even about Italian take-away options. I wasn't really sure what it was about. 'I was doing it, the account's in my name, just let me pay for it.'

Suddenly he turned round and for the first time ever he properly snapped at me. It made me flinch. 'You don't have to pay for it. I don't need you to pay for everything.'

I felt stung. 'I'm not paying for everything.' *And even if I were, is that something to get the arse about?* 'It just makes sense for me to pay a bit more for things than you while –'

'– While I'm not working. I know, I'm not working. Thanks for bringing it up. I hadn't noticed. So I'm not working and yet I'm suggesting extravagant takeaways. Fine.'

I was outraged at the injustice. 'I didn't say that. I didn't even think that. And when I said you're not working, I didn't mean it that way, I didn't mean it in any way, it's just a fact. And it's fine, we can cope, you're going to get something else. In the meantime we're OK.' I paused, swallowing back an odd lump in my throat. 'We're fine.'

I think he heard my tone change, heard the slight wobble in my voice. Suddenly his frustration seeped from him and instead he was sheepish and quiet. He ran a hand through his hair and sighed.

'I'm sorry, Soph. I'm so sorry. I didn't mean to snap. I'm an idiot. It's just I didn't expect moving in together to be like this.'

Shit, what did he mean by that? I felt the panic rise in my chest. I was really happy, happier than I'd ever been. Wasn't he? I think he saw the look in my eyes, and suddenly he was stroking my arms, pulling me closer.

'No, Soph. That's not what I meant.' He swore under his breath. 'I just meant, when we moved in together I never expected that I wouldn't be able to pull my own weight, that you'd have to carry me.'

I was confused and not a little irritated. 'I'm not carrying you. We're carrying each other.'

He shook his head. 'Not at the moment we aren't, sweetheart. You're carrying me. And it's lovely that you want to, I'm bloody lucky that you can, but it makes me frustrated. It feels wrong.'

I shook my head in annoyance. 'We're a partnership. We share stuff. When you're working you earn considerably more than me. You might not be working now but that's going to change soon enough and we'll be back to the usual dynamic. This is just a temporary thing. It's certainly not something to feel awkward about.'

'But I do. It doesn't feel right.' He could tell I was

getting annoyed, but he said it anyway. I had to give him points for honesty.

'You know you're an idiot? That this is ridiculous?'

He nodded sombrely. 'I know. I do. And I'm sorry for being a twat about it. But it bothers me.' He paused for a minute before waggling a finger in my direction. 'But don't pretend when it was the other way round that you didn't feel awkward about it. Remember the meals out where you insisted on splitting the bill and the phase where you'd make sure you booked the cinema tickets and whatever else to "make up" for it if by some miracle you did let me pay the full amount for a dinner?' He made speech marks with his fingers for 'make up'. It made me want to bite them in annoyance.

He was right. But that wasn't the point.

'I got over it.' It was almost true.

He grinned at me. 'I know. And I know this is a ridiculous row.'

I nodded. 'It's really stupid. Especially since it's somewhat academic – it's all our shared money anyway.'

He took the tablet away again and began putting in his details. 'Let me use some of our savings to buy us dinner.'

I couldn't help but smile. 'Fine, but for the record, being funny about me earning more than you, even temporarily, is a bit lame. I thought better of you.'

'I know. I'm a terrible feminist.'

Git.

Even with the moments of bickering and the strain of Adam's job situation, we continued to have a lot of sex.

Maybe it was our matching (and rather enthusiastic) libidos, but the fact that most days ended with a cuddle and some kind of rude fun meant we stayed emotionally close even with the day-to-day difficulties. It's really hard to be pissed off with someone if you're falling asleep with your legs tangled together and his arms round you – although his occasional duvet hogging remained a hard limit.

That said, there came a point where suddenly things didn't feel so solid any more. And it came, much to my surprise, from the sexual, and even submissive, side of things rather than any awkwardness about money or any real-life concerns. It was also, mostly, all in my head.

The thing about boundaries shifting is that sometimes you don't feel you've gone too far until it's too late to come back. I know it sounds a bit fortune-cookie-wisdom-ish, but it is definitely true. Unfortunately, and somewhat inevitably, it was a conclusion I came to after the event.

Adam had pushed my boundaries and buttons in dozens, if not hundreds, of different ways in the time we had been together. He'd hurt me, embarrassed me, aroused me, in ways I'd never have dreamed of, and in some cases not even have considered erotic until he did them. I was in his thrall. It was as exciting as it was surprising, and for someone who enjoys being on the back foot as a fundamental part of her submission, it was a very heady thing. I loved it. Loved the psychology of the things we got up to. Loved how, when it was over, we'd make dinner together or watch telly or hang the washing – quiet moments that were such a mundane and steady contrast to the filth that had gone before.

Over time I began to get used to his mind fuckery, his

ability to keep me on the back foot by laying the ground work for an experience we would have together long before we did it. Sometimes (but, to my frustration, still only sometimes) I would be able to silence the curiosity and the nerves that he tried to build. OK, who am I kidding? I couldn't silence them, but I could certainly quieten them. But then sometimes he could see me becoming blasé, and that's when he upped the stakes more, the clash of our dominance and submission suddenly becoming more competitive than our computer gaming (which once got so bad Adam chucked his controller on the floor in frustration – I laughed, he kissed me, we got distracted).

To start with I didn't realise what a challenge he had in store for me. He had decided, after some soul-searching, that perhaps the best way to guarantee work was to set up as a freelance copywriter from home. He'd begun scouting for clients for his fledgling agency and when he was recommended to a large company in York by an ex-colleague, he was invited up to pitch some ideas for a brochure and advertising campaign. He asked if I fancied making the trip up with him. Never averse to some time meandering the snickelways, I agreed, and the next thing I knew he'd thrown caution to the wind and booked a posh hotel suite for the weekend, happy that he could claim it back on expenses, and I was Googling nice places to have dinner once he'd completed his meetings.

He'd warned me the week before that he was going to push my boundaries further than ever before while we were away. I felt the prickle of nerves, of course – I'm not daft – but I have to admit that I was feeling a little complacent. Everything he had pushed me with before I had coped with (for the most part), so while I had a flutter of nerves, it was mostly in fear of letting him down rather than worrying what he was up to. Stupid Sophie.

The suite was gorgeous, with views of the river from every window, a massive claw-footed bath and a bed big enough for six (or at least for me, doing my very best star-fish, and Adam, which was quite enough). Adam went off for his meeting while I wandered around the shops and had a leisurely lunch. We agreed we would meet back at the hotel in the late afternoon for, I assumed, some kind of sexual shenanigans before we went for dinner.

That was the first time I underestimated him that afternoon. Unfortunately it wasn't the last.

No one can see me this far up. That's what I kept telling myself as the sun warmed my bare skin. Even if someone on one of the tourist charters puttering past far below caught a glimpse of me, they'd probably just think I was admiring the view of the river. Unmoving. For half an hour. And they were moving. They wouldn't be able to tell. *Unless they came back. What if they came back?*

Adam had been subtle, after all; the rope securing my wrists to the top of the balcony was as long as it needed to be and no more, stretching my arms wide and allowing me to lean down and hide my predicament by pressing my bare breasts against what had started as cool metal, but which had warmed up the longer I stayed out there. I suppose I should have been grateful that the balcony was child-proof and as such there were few gaps for any passers-by to see how little I was wearing. He was defin-itely testing my patience. He'd warned me not to look, no matter how big the temptation or how bored I was, and while the sound of him moving around the suite, doors opening and closing, even the TV channel changing, gave me some idea of what was going on, the temptation to turn my head was high. I 'casually' flicked my hair off my shoulder, risking a glance only to find that the depth of the balcony meant I could see very little; I was unable to turn with my wrists immobilised.

And it wasn't just my arms he'd secured. My ankles were anchored to the struts that held the balcony in place. He'd spread my legs just a little further than was comfortable, leaving me with a twinge in my thigh muscles. Adam enjoyed that, enjoyed my reaction as I realised I would effectively be trapped here until he decided otherwise. My foot flexed even as he knelt down to tie it, betraying the nerves that made me want to bolt, to kick away, before the feel of his hand, gently stroking my thigh, calmed me as though I were a spooked animal.

I tried desperately to be rational. I trusted him. I knew he had no more interest in doing anything public than I did, that we enjoyed our shared secret. Suddenly all the research into hotels he'd done made sense. Even while I was nervous and awkward, I knew it must be safe and discreet, even if it felt like he was displaying me to anyone who happened past.

Adam ran his hands over me possessively, pushing back a strand of hair, brushing a bit of fluff from my arse. The nerves came back a little when, having ensured I wasn't going anywhere, he disappeared off, returning with one of his favourite combinations: the glass butt plug and that bloody inflatable plug. As he pushed the glass inside me I whimpered a bit, forgetting myself and where I was. I flushed red and ducked my head into my shoulder for a moment – daft, really, as if there *were* anyone in eyeshot it would hardly stop them seeing me. When he slid the inflatable plug into my cunt, he chuckled to himself at how wet I already was. I steeled myself, biting my lip to silence the moans as he pressed the bulb and inflated the plug, filling me. He moved beside me, leaning casually with his back against the balcony railing, looking at my face, watching my teeth press harder against my lip, seeing my nostrils flare every time he pressed the button and filled me further. He kept pressing, smiling at me for a second, until he saw real grumpiness on my face.

'No, *no*. You don't give me that look if I want to do this to you.'

His tone was sharp. I had, as ever, no clue what *that look* was or how I could stop it, but his displeasure made me regretful. I felt a little worried, too, but I was mainly upset at disappointing him, displeasing him. I tripped over my words as I replied.

'I'm sorry, there's no look, I'm not *looking*, I just . . .' I tailed off in uncertainty, frustrated as ever at how, despite words being my thing, he could leave me so inarticulate. So unsure. My voice was small. 'I want to be good.'

His smile made my stomach flip. He leaned down and kissed my shoulder. 'I know you do. And mostly you're a *very* good girl. You do please me.' As the words filtered into my brain they were punctuated with three more hisses of that bloody plug. 'Best make sure that's nice and tight.' He grinned at me. Even though my cunt was already so full – it felt like his fist was in there – even though I was aching already, I smiled back, enjoying the giddy look he gets sometimes when we play, like a little kid let lose in a sweet shop. A smutty, evil kid, admittedly.

He really was adamant that everything stay nice and tight. His final piece of rope tied both plugs tightly in place, leaving a jaunty bow on my hip. As he stood up, brushing dust from his trousers, he picked up the little box which made the plug vibrate. I moaned quietly in the back of my throat, a plea almost. He kissed my side.

'Don't worry. I'm not going to put it on high. I know it'll be hard to be quiet coming out here. I just want to have it working enough to keep you ticking over.'

I snorted at his wording as well as the sentiment. Tied, naked, plugged and awaiting his pleasure? As if keeping me aroused was going to be a problem. The vibrations burst into life inside me and the trembling in my legs began. He kissed my shoulder.

'Do you trust me my Sophie?' His expression was searching. I nodded, certain.

'Yes. I do.' He looked at me for a couple more seconds before nodding his approval.

'Good. Just remember, if you trust me no real harm will come to you.' I tried not to shiver at the warning in his words. 'Now remember, keep looking straight ahead and be a good girl for me.'

I smiled. 'I promise.'

He went inside again. I watched the boats far below, a man walking his dog on the riverbank. There was nothing else to do, just stand, wait, and enjoy the view and the unseasonably warm weather. As I stood there, that feeling of submissive simplicity kicked in. I trusted him. Loved him. I wanted to please him. I knew he wouldn't do anything to harm me. He was clearly inside plotting something, but it didn't matter what. I could cope with whatever he threw at me. I was already wet in anticipation. My eyes grew a little sleepy, enjoying the warmth of the sunshine.

In hindsight, I realise he'd lulled me into a false sense of security.

I don't know how long I'd been out there before he came out to untie me. His voice was low as he began undoing the knots, telling me to stay looking ahead, not to move even when I could do so. I flexed my wrists a little once he had undone them, but otherwise stayed in position as he reached down to my ankles.

He tutted loudly, running his fingers along my sticky inner thighs as he went. I restrained the urge to point out that when you're left standing upright with something vibrating between your legs for a significant length of time it's unreasonable not to expect gravity to work its magic. He was in a stern-looking mood and even I'm not that foolhardy.

Once he'd untied me he put his hands over my eyes.

'I'm going to lead you inside now, but I want you to keep your eyes shut. Do you understand?'

I said yes. Suddenly I didn't feel quite as confident as I had before.

'Good girl.' It was one of his favoured terms of affection, and made me feel a little comforted. Not much, but a bit. And every little helps, right?

As he led me back inside, he put a blindfold over my eyes. His hands held my wrists behind my back and suddenly he was pushing me to the floor.

'Kneel.'

I knelt, slowly, unsure of where in the room I was. My knees made contact with a fluffy rug which I knew was in the centre of the room. I sank into it, taking a crumb of comfort from the warmth and the softness of it, even as Adam began to tie my wrists behind me. His silence was making me nervous, as was the blindfold, which he pulled slightly lower on my nose.

'Can you see anything?'

I opened my mouth to speak but before I could do so he slapped me hard across my face. The surprise of it (and the not-inconsiderable force) made me gasp. He laughed quietly, and the sound made me feel nervous. 'I guess not.'

I sat very still, half expecting him to hit me again, wondering where the blow would come from. But then he was gone.

I could hear him moving around. Sometimes he was nearby, sometimes in the bedroom. At one point it even sounded like he was in the en suite. I had no idea what he was doing, and not being on home turf meant it was much harder to mentally picture where he was, let alone know what he was up to. The carpet that flowed through great parts of the apartment masked the sound of his movement. I was constantly jumping, wondering if every slight creak and change in the air was him coming closer.

Finally he stroked my face. I flinched, half expecting him to slap me again, but his hand was warm and soothing. It was comforting, a return of *my* Adam, and that connection made me feel a little calmer for a moment. Until he spoke, at least.

'Do you remember your safe word?'

For fuck's sake. I sighed, in nervousness I think, my tone brusque. 'Yes.'

He leaned in and his voice was steely enough to make me shiver. 'Don't take that tone. Just remember it in case you need to use it.'

I felt a surge of fury. I opened my mouth to retort, thought better of it and harrumphed to myself instead (that's a bit better, right?). At that point I don't think it mattered. He was gone. I think.

I don't know how long I knelt there. It was long enough to begin to feel a little uncomfortable. I wanted to shuffle a little on the floor, but had no way of knowing whether he was watching me or not, and no intention of showing him I was uncomfortable if he was in the room.

Suddenly I heard a whoosh and felt a sting on my breast. The cane. Fuck.

I hate the cane. It hurts more than anything else he uses on me – there's little room for tone with it. With a flogger, if you use it gently, it can be really sensual, little more than a tickle. Even at its lightest, the cane makes me shiver. This wasn't anywhere near its lightest.

He hit my breast twice and then seemed to move behind me – it was hard to tell because of the rug. He hit my arse. The noise of the cane slicing through the air made me wince, but there was never time to prepare for it even if I knew where it was going to land. Suddenly there were lines of fire all over my body. He was relentless. I tried not to cry out, but the pain felt intense, and not being able to see him made me feel oddly bereft.

He hit me a lot, enough that I began to whimper under my breath. It was a harsh kind of pain, and despite the vibrations in my cunt, I struggled to cope with it, feeling myself tear up behind the blindfold as the relentless lashes continued. Surely he would be getting bored now?

No such luck. Every so often he paused and I felt him move closer. At one point he ran a fingernail across several marks he'd made on my breast and the pain made me cry out. He put his finger to my mouth, mocking me as he whispered 'sssssssshhhh' into my ear.

I was two people in conflict. The rational side of me knew this was a head fuck, knew he was messing with me, knew this was intense, as intense as he had warned me it would be, but that fundamentally this was my lovely boyfriend Adam, who I could trust and who would look out for me. My more irrational side was in a panic, reacting only to the pain, adrenaline and nerves, desperately hoping it would soon be over and that we would move on to something that was slightly less challenging. Which side was going to win out? No bloody clue. But for the first time in a long time it was a balanced battle.

Finally, thankfully, he stopped. I heard the sound of him throwing the cane on the sofa. It was all I could do not to collapse on the floor in relief.

I felt him move nearer. He grabbed the back of my head and pushed me forward, and I realised I was nuzzling his crotch through his trousers. I leaned into him, eager, probably pathetically so. I rubbed my face against him, feeling him harden against me. I opened my mouth, a silent but fairly obvious indication of where I wanted things to go. He patted my head.

'Not yet, in a minute.'

I felt a surge of disappointment as he grabbed me by the arms and lifted me to my wobbly feet. I heard him pick up the control box and bulb for the plug, which was still deep inside me. It was just as well, as I think otherwise I'd have fallen over them. He led me into the bedroom. I didn't even have time to feel relief, as he led me straight through; suddenly the cold tiles of the bathroom floor were under my feet. This was unexpected.

His voice was brusque. 'Into the bath.'

I clambered in tentatively, using my feet to get my bearings. My lack of sight and my hands being tied behind my back made me unbalanced and ungainly. I was relieved to find the bath was empty; my first fleeting thought was that we would be doing some kind of water breath play, and the idea of doing that without the reassurance of eye contact made me feel real fear.

It was OK, though. The bath was wide enough that I could kneel comfortably in the bottom, waiting for whatever happened next. I heard him unzip his fly near my head somewhere and for a moment I thought I was finally going to get to taste him – maybe he had moved me to the bath because he wanted to come across my body and was worried about getting it everywhere.

But that wasn't what happened. Two things happened almost simultaneously. The plug in my cunt burst into high-speed vibrations which, bearing in mind the eroticism of everything that had happened before, meant I felt my orgasm thundering towards me like a steam train.

And Adam began to piss on me.

The warm stream started across my breasts. I froze. My

brain pretty much shorted out. As my orgasm built inexorably, the stream moved up, nearer my shoulders, wetting my hair. I began to shudder, partly from my orgasm and partly from shock. I came, but my cries were distressed. How could he have done that? We'd always said that was a hard limit. How could he have done that? I felt grief, bone-deep disappointment. I wanted to cry, I wanted to punch him, but I couldn't do anything, I was scared my legs wouldn't support me if I tried to move. The sound of my orgasm had shifted to a muted series of sobs.

Adam's hands were at my waist. Stilling the vibrations, untying the rope that kept the plugs in place, pulling them out. Suddenly there was a flash of light, the blindfold had been taken off and I was staring right at him, his brown eyes wide with concern. I blinked, trying to focus on him, trying to focus on anything, realising I couldn't because my eyes were full of tears.

He was talking to me, but I didn't understand what he was saying for a few seconds. He kept repeating himself, as he leaned round, pulling the ropes from my wrists, helping me up, grabbing a warm towel from the rail.

'Sophie? It was water. It was warm water. Just warm water.'

I blinked at him, trying to understand, my brain not quite working. He held up a glass. 'It's water. I dribbled it on you with my mouth.'

I nodded. He smiled in relief, pleased that I understood, pleased that I knew the extent of his head fuck now. He kissed my face, pushing my wet hair over my shoulder. Wet from water.

'Oh, sweetheart, you were amazing. Are you OK?' He

kissed me again, pressing kisses to my face, rubbing my arms, which were suddenly cold with goosebumps. 'You're freezing, come on, let's get you into bed for a minute.'

He half-led, half-carried me back into the bedroom and we clambered into bed together. The warmth of his body and the duvet he covered me with helped me back to myself a little. He stroked my back, pressing kisses to me, hugging me. He was my Adam, back once more.

We kissed. We gently made love. It was slow and tender and affectionate, a chance for us to reconnect, for me to regain my equilibrium. He moved slowly above me, his hand between my thighs, touching my clit, bringing about an orgasm we shared together, one I gave willingly rather than having it wrenched from me.

As our breathing slowed we lay quietly together in the warmth, mindful that we had time before our dinner reservations for a bit of recovery.

I looked at my breasts and thighs, curious to see the marks of the cane. There were none. He sleepily told me he'd used it, but not enough to mark – it had just felt more intense because of the way he had messed with my mind along the way. I couldn't argue. It had felt intense. It had all felt intense.

'I really thought you had . . .' My voice was tentative to start with and trailed off before I could form the words.

He stroked my face and pressed a kiss to my lips. 'I know, sweetheart. I thought you had understood when I talked about no real harm coming to you. When I saw you start to shake I knew you hadn't.' He kissed me again. 'I'm so sorry if it all felt too much.'

I wrapped my arms around him. 'It's alright, I'm OK.

I just didn't understand what you meant by "real" harm in the heat of everything going on. I got caught up in things.'

He looked at my closely. 'But you're OK? Promise?'

I smiled at him and nodded. 'I'm OK. Promise.' It was the first time I had lied to him.

I still couldn't quite believe it. He hadn't pissed on me, he hadn't pushed past my hard limits. The relief was immense. I could still trust him. But as I lay there listening to his breathing as he dozed, tears began to fall down my face. There was one problem.

I couldn't trust myself.

Chapter Thirteen

It's ironic, really, that something that *didn't* happen could have had such a massive impact on my mindset. But it really did.

I had to hand it to Adam. He'd said he was going to mess with my mind and he did that to grand effect. And he was lovely afterwards, really lovely. He knew how much it affected me and took great pains to reassure me. He was, in terms of aftercare, a good and responsible dominant. But more than that, as my boyfriend he was loving and caring and concerned.

That evening I lay there wide-eyed, my brain whirring, while he dozed. Then we went out for a decadent dinner, all beautifully cooked seafood and the kind of sinful chocolate pudding that makes me swoon. He complimented me on my dress and my throat went dry at the sight of him in one of the sharpest of his suits. It was romantic, fun, and Adam was on great form. We were as comfortable around each other as ever before. It was lovely, genuinely so.

The problem was, even while I was enjoying the evening, there was a tiny part of my brain having a freak-out. It was like an alternate track: mostly I could ignore it, but every so often it would get louder and then I was thinking again about something I didn't want to think about at all.

And then we went back to the suite. We snuck out onto the balcony on hands and knees so no one could see us and, giggling like children, laid naked on the ground, just a spare blanket nabbed from the wardrobe keeping us from the cold of the concrete. We snuggled together to minimise the chill, and then snuggling turned to groping and then we were fucking, laughing about how uncomfortable it was to be on top (the concrete was hard on the knees) and taking our pleasure from each other. As we recovered from our respective orgasms, we cuddled together to watch the stars and then he kissed me and told me he loved me and I kissed him back and told him I loved him too.

It was a really memorable night, beautiful and romantic – well, as beautiful and romantic as it could be when earlier on I was convinced Adam had pissed on me. But that was the problem. I should have been able to shake off the odd feeling, but I really couldn't. And to be fair to him, it wasn't about Adam, it was about me.

As I lay in bed, my mind kept going back to the moment in the bath, the building orgasm, the certainty that he was pissing on me. Two things kept going round in my head.

1. I thought he was pissing on me and I didn't stop him.
2. I thought he was pissing on me and I came anyway.

I know some people enjoy the taboo, but watersports had always been a hard limit for me. Despite my limits shifting during the time I was with Adam, certain things remained out of bounds. All the illegal stuff, obviously, anything likely to cause permanent injury or damage, anything toilet related, anything involving multiple partners (yes, even though I'd had a threesome before I was wary about ballsing up a relationship by having a threesome while in one), anything involving needles (I'm a big wuss). I trusted him to keep to those limits and, really, he had kept to them.

I hadn't.

I felt confused by my inaction. Self-disgusted and gutless too. Often, in the aftermath of sexual play, I get little flashbacks to what has happened, the things we've done. The more challenging something is, the more likely that is to happen. In my earliest D/s experiences it was this thought process that helped me come to terms with the thoughts and feelings that were elicited by my kinky new experiences. It was both hot and helpful in allowing me to come to understand the emotional side of what I was doing, what I was allowing to be done to me.

But the problem with this was, the more I thought about it, the more disconnected I felt. Even the most challenging and painful D/s I had ever indulged in had, fundamentally, been fun. Challenging, yes, often embarrassing (but I think it's pretty obvious by now that I like that on some twisted level). But this was different. Adam's intentions had been good – evil, but good: the erotic equivalent of scaring yourself shitless at a house of horrors and coming out the other end unscathed, giggling and with your heart beating with fear at a scenario that was only really ever in your head. But I couldn't shake it off and discount it that way.

I knew I didn't use my safe word enough, even when things were intense to the point of feeling unbearable. Hell, two of the four times I'd ever used it were because

I got cramp in my foot while tied up and thus felt the need to hop around shaking my leg to try and get the blood flowing again (I know, it's an alluring image).

Rationally I knew it wasn't right to see using my safe word as a 'failure' but somewhere in my head it felt a little like it was – or if not a failure then a defeat, waving the white flag. Normally that was fine, because the people I was with factored my stubborn bloody-mindedness into their treatment of me, but here, here the responsibility had been mine, and I'd abdicated it. I'd frozen.

I tried to rationalise it. I was shocked. It all happened really quickly. Somewhere in the back of my mind I knew Adam hadn't been pissing on me – maybe I could tell by the lack of smell or the fact the water wasn't too hot or . . . but it just felt odd. I felt really out of sorts, and it lasted for several weeks.

Adam and I talked about it; he knew me well and could tell that things weren't quite right, but I deliberately spoke lightly of it when we spoke of it at all. I brushed aside his repeated apologies because I honestly believed he had nothing to apologise for, the responsibility had been mine. His reassurance, his kindness, made me love him all the more. He cuddled me, stroked my hair, talked it through. I think he thought we were through it and it was OK. But despite us going back to our day-to-day lives – working, fucking, bickering about the news, watching TV, seeing friends and family – the experience cast an oddly long shadow over my mood and kept popping into my head in quiet moments.

It also made me question how far D/s could go. Shifting boundaries are natural, but how far is too far? Suddenly my frustration with James, who had been unable to continue hurting me because he had pushed beyond the limits of what he considered acceptable and safe and kind, seemed a bit unfair. The situations were different, but the similarities gave me pause. For the first time in months he was on my mind again. That felt weird too.

Of course, seeing James felt even weirder than thinking about him.

By this point it had been almost a year since our last meeting. We'd gone for a rather half-hearted lunch which, at the time, I had hoped might encourage a reconciliation, but instead was the last in a series of ever-more-impersonal meetings and communications which then tailed off into silence.

The last unreturned message was mine. I'd decided that it was too difficult living in a land of ifs and maybes, so I'd taken the initiative to step back – if you can call disappearing into a pit of mopey despair taking initiative. The fact he hadn't tried to contact me again vindicated my response.

I'd moved on.

But, of course, when I saw him next I was momentarily brought up short. I was in the pub with a few colleagues after work celebrating someone's birthday, when I saw someone who looked like him standing at the bar. This 'recognition' of what turned out to be strangers was something that had happened a lot in the early months following the break-up of our unusual relationship. Over time it had stopped, but something about this guy – the haircut, the way he held himself, maybe the cut of his suit – brought James back to my mind. Hell, maybe it was just the fact I'd been thinking about him a lot recently, in light of what, in my head, I referred to as Weegate. I know, it's a ridiculous name, but branding it that made me laugh, and I was trying to make the whole episode feel less portentous. Of course, one silly name isn't going to do that all on its own, and in the pensive moments when it still popped into my head I began to wonder – in light of how it had affected me – if I'd been fair in how I'd tried to help James through his concerns about what we were doing together.

I stared at the man at the bar long enough that Mark, our local government reporter and the guy I sat next to at work, elbowed me in the ribs. 'You all right there, Soph? You look like you're about to start dribbling.'

I let myself be dragged back into the conversation. 'Nah, I wasn't leching. He's not my type. I just thought he was someone I knew.'

Shona, our news editor and the bluntest woman I've ever met, turned to look at him. 'He's someone I wish I knew. Nice bum. Suit looks good on him too, looks expensive. I bet he'd be OK with buying a round of drinks every now and then as well.' She looked meaningfully at Mark, who sighed.

'You're subtle, but I believe it's my turn to go to the bar. Help me carry, Soph?'

I nodded absently and began to shuffle along the wooden booth to get up. That was when he turned round.

It was like he knew we were talking about him – although we weren't talking loudly and even Shona was a few drinks away from her loud and rowdy best. His eyes met mine and the flicker of recognition shifted to surprise. He smiled and waved.

Shit.

Shona cackled. 'Well if he isn't someone you know then he's certainly keen to meet you. He definitely looks better from the front. Is he single?'

The words were harder to say than they should have been. 'I don't know.'

I am a chicken. I waved at him and then walked past to go to the loo, hoping against hope that he'd have been served and moved away before I had to help Mark bring the drinks back to the table.

No such luck. He was pretty much loitering outside the loo, waiting for me.

'Hi, Sophie.'

'Hello.'

'How are you? It's been ages. You're looking well.'

'Thanks. I'm good, really good. You?' The small talk felt ridiculous and made me want to run away. I suppose it was a small step forward that I mostly felt skin-crawling awkwardness rather than any surge of lust. Although I couldn't help but notice that his hair still fell over his face – I could never resist reaching up to brush it away. I put my hand in my pocket.

The silence lengthened. Were we done? I was hoping we were done.

He cleared his throat and gestured to a table behind him. 'So. I'm with some work colleagues, I should probably go back. They probably think I'm trying to pick you up or something . . .' He laughed and I restrained the urge to kick him in the shins. Was it so unreasonable for folk to think that he'd be trying to pick me up? And, hold on, why did I care? I didn't *want* him to pick me up. Right? God, this was confusing. I thought of Adam – simple, straightforward, I-know-what-he's-thinking Adam – and remembered I didn't need to do this any more. The thought made me smile. It grounded me somehow.

'I'm with people too. I should go. Glad you're well.'

'You too. We should meet for a drink soon.'

I brushed him off with a casual 'yeah', knowing he wouldn't ever in a million years get round to calling, and fled to grab a couple of pints off Mark, with James's farewell ringing in my ears.

He emailed me at work the following day, asking me when I wanted that drink.

I literally didn't know what to say. A straight out 'no' seemed quite abrupt, while an 'I'm seeing someone' seemed a bit like gloating and made it sound like I'd assumed he was asking me out romantically, which was quite a leap bearing in mind how things had ended. I didn't want to go out with him for drinks, though, which had to be progress, so in the end I just ignored the mail, sure he'd forget about it in a day or two.

He didn't.

That Friday I'd arranged to meet Charlotte for drinks after work. She'd been working in town for the day and we thought we'd take advantage of that fact, and happy hour, to get a chance to catch up. I was a little wary about it – I'd not spent much time with her since Adam and I had started seeing each other seriously, and was a little worried she'd try and start a conversation about his (redoubtable) sexual prowess that would make me want to flee. Or get drunk. Actually, that could work fine.

Shortly before I was due to leave the office I got called down to reception to sign for a massive bunch of flowers, all cellophane and ribbon and green bits. I felt a bit sheepish carrying it upstairs to my desk, but I couldn't help smiling to myself. As Shona flapped around me, smelling the lilies that formed the centre of the bouquet, I opened the card.

How about that drink? – James x

My jaw dropped open and I pushed the gift card back into the envelope and shoved it in my pocket. Shona began to laugh as she saw my expression.

'Is Adam sending rude messages to you at work?'

I laughed in spite of myself. 'Chance would be a fine thing.' That was, of course, a fib, but it probably wasn't the wisest thing to admit to my news editor that some mornings when I looked like I was earnestly replying to my emails I was actually discussing what was going to happen when we reconvened in our living room later that night.

I got my head down and finished typing up some council meeting report information, hoping the tell-tale blush on my cheeks was going down. One thing was for sure: it was fairly obvious now that I needed to formally say 'no thanks' to that drink.

I decided the easiest way was to email. I know, a bit gutless maybe, but in my defence we'd not had the best track record of phone conversations. Or talking in person, actually. It seemed safest. Still pretty awkward, all things considered, but safest.

I know it was blunt. I wrote and rewrote it a dozen times,
but I didn't want to write anything that inadvertently made
it sound like I wished I was free for drinks with him, or
that I actively didn't want to see him. Also, I didn't want it
to sound like somehow Adam curtailed my social life if
James was just angling for an innocent catch-up (although
I'm pretty sure it wasn't – they were a pretty swanky bunch
of flowers).

James hadn't replied by the time I left work. I wasn't
sure he would. It's hardly as if he was going to start asking
extended questions about my love life. I hurried to meet
Charlotte, keen to kick-start the weekend.

Charlotte was on good form. From the moment she
burst into the bar, pulling off the hat that had been pro-
tecting her hair from the rain and using her fingers to
comb out her curls as she read the cocktail menu, she
chatted cheerfully about anything and everything. She
seemed really happy.

Surprisingly so in fact, bearing in mind the chats I'd had
with Tom. A few cocktails in I decided to risk asking her
how things were going. I was pretty sure she wasn't putting
a brave face on anything, but at the same time it seemed
somewhat surreal that she was happy and he had been so

down. Unless something had changed fundamentally in the last few weeks.

Definitely time to start prodding. I know it sounds nosey. But it's not nosiness, it's curiosity, remember?

'So, how are things going with you and Tom?'

I'll concede, as lines of questioning go, it was something of a blunt instrument, but I was three cocktails down myself by this point and not exactly the most insightful interviewer. That said, even I didn't expect the conversation to move quite the way it did.

'Brilliant. Yeah, he's amazing. Not last weekend, the weekend before, he arranged a threesome with a girl that we met at a munch. She dominated me, he dominated both of us.' A smile played across her lips. 'It was intense. Really intense. Quite challenging. It reminded me of you, actually.'

I was momentarily confused. 'I'm intense and challenging?'

My hand was resting on the table. She tapped it gently, although I couldn't tell if it was in rebuke or a kind of affection.

'No, it reminded me of dominating you.'

I blushed.

It had happened not long before I met James. I have no regrets about it, but the experience was one of the catalysts that made me realise that I wanted a romantic D/s relationship rather than a dom with benefits. Thomas had met Charlotte before and then we all met at what remained my first and only munch. We got on very well, with a fair amount of flirtation on either side, and then, one memorable bank holiday weekend, we ended up having a threesome. She made me rim her – OK, to start with she *made me*, but then I did it willingly – and she used the cane on me. They wrote on me and then fucked lying next to me. It was intense, with lots of rising emotion, lots of pain and humiliation, and at the time it was one of the most amazing sexual experiences I'd had, albeit one I wasn't sure I wanted to have again.

Suddenly I was the one smiling, albeit slightly sheepishly. She stroked my hand with her fingertips, before picking up her cocktail.

'It's funny. Before that weekend with you and Tom I hadn't ever switched before. I thought I might be interested in trying but I didn't think it was something I would naturally have a flair for, as it were.'

I smiled at her wryly. 'In the nicest possible way, love, I'd beg to differ. You were a natural bitch.'

'Bitch or switch?'

'Both. Definitely both.'

She laughed, and two guys at the table next to us turned to look at her, not that she noticed. Charlotte might have been stunning but she didn't care about it in the least, and that carefree nature was one of the things I admired about her.

She nodded. 'I was quite mean to you, wasn't I?'

I rolled my eyes. 'You think?'

She grinned. 'It was just so much fun, though, seeing how you reacted, trying to predict what you were going to do next and figure out how to make you do what I wanted you to do. I'd not appreciated the psychological side of topping before until I did it with you. It was brilliant, I really enjoyed it.'

The silence lengthened for a bit. It was one of those

moments when the conversation could go one of two ways. I could change the subject, or I could express some interest and she would continue. Did it feel awkward? A bit, but not too much – Thomas and I hadn't slept together for a long time, and even then there had been no jealousy there. I had to admit my overriding emotion was burning curiosity. In for a penny, in for a pound. 'You enjoyed it, but I can hear a '"but" coming in here somewhere.'

She nodded.

'There were points where I was wondering what it would be like if it was me, being made to do the things you were made to do. Being written on, hurt.' I felt myself getting a bit warm thinking about it. I swallowed and nodded, suddenly incapable of speech, my brain slowed by X-rated thoughts.

'So I told Tom I was curious. That I wanted to have a threesome where basically I was *you*, dominated by them both. And he got chatting to this girl, Jo, at a munch. Really good laugh, friendly, very sexy, long dark hair and green eyes. We went out for some drinks so we were sure we'd all get on and then he arranged it all.'

Her eyes were shining with energy and remembered excitement. 'He arranged it all for me.'

Her voice had got quieter, and I leaned in to listen. 'I didn't know exactly when it was going to happen, just that it was. When he first tied me up and blindfolded me in his living room on Saturday night I thought it was just the two of us doing stuff. And then the doorbell rang and he went to answer it.'

'Did you guess it was her?'

For a moment her face looked shy. 'Not to start with. I

thought it was someone selling something or he was somehow messing with my head. And then I heard who-ever it was walk in and the murmur of voices got louder and I realised –'

I finished her sentence for her. 'He was *really* messing with your head.'

She laughed and continued. 'She didn't speak to me when she walked in, but she began touching me. Not sex-ually, just matter-of-factly. It was like she was assessing me, pinching me, squeezing and prodding, running her hands over me like she was checking out a piece of meat.'

My throat suddenly felt a little dry. 'How did that make you feel?'

'Horrible. Awkward. Embarrassed. Humiliated.' Char-lotte smiled at me wryly. 'Incredible. It was so fucking hot.'

I smiled back. 'Ah yes. Always that awkward mixture.'

Charlotte nodded and leaned forward to clink her glass with mine. 'Sometimes it's nice to know it's not just me who feels that. It was really challenging. She was relentless, she hit me all over with a ruler.' Charlotte's face turned to mock outrage. 'It really bloody hurt. I ended up covered in these little square red marks from the end of it.'

I had a mental image of her pale skin marked that way. I have to admit the thought of it made me squirm a little. I definitely wasn't interested in having sex with anyone but Adam right now, but, remembering the soft paleness of her skin, I felt intrigued at the thought of the marks.

'She and Tom chatted as she went, about how well I bruised, the sort of pain I'd taken before, whether I enjoyed it, what he enjoyed hitting me with. Even as she was hitting me I wasn't really her focus, I felt like a play-thing, a toy, something to do while she chatted with him. It was so demeaning and so hot. I totally got why you enjoyed it. And then they fucked and I watched, and it was everything I hoped for. She told me I should thank her for fucking him in front of me, and I did. It was just so much fun. It was such an amazing thing for him to arrange, everything I'd fantasised about and more.'

I smiled, understanding completely her wonder at the intensity of it, and relieved at her obvious affection for Thomas having organised it. I did have one question, though. 'So, I'm intrigued.'

She laughed. 'Ask away, Soph, I think we're past the polite chit-chat.'

I grinned. 'For the record, this is *much* more fun than polite chit-chat. But I'm curious. Did you feel jealous or weird watching Tom fuck her?'

Charlotte didn't hesitate before she replied. 'Not at all. Let's face it, Tom and I aren't dating. We're not into each other that way. We have an arrangement similar to the one you had with him. It's a lot of fun. He's not my boyfriend. I don't want him to be. And he doesn't want a girlfriend.'

I feigned a sudden, in-depth interest in the drinks menu. Ouch. Poor Tom. I thought it was time to change the subject, mostly by getting more drinks.

The rest of the evening passed quickly. Charlotte and I nattered about work, she told me once more she had never seen Adam so smitten (which still made me grin), we bickered about what to see at the cinema the following Saturday when we'd all agreed to go out. It was fun, exactly the kind of Friday night you needed after a long week at work.

It had seemed a waste leaving James's flowers at work but I didn't want to bring them home either – I'm no etiquette expert but it seemed like that would be pretty bad form, potentially made worse by the fact they looked incredibly expensive and Adam was still worried about his finances. Instead I gave them to Charlotte when we staggered our separate ways. As far as I was concerned things were done with James. I thought of mentioning to Adam that he'd been in touch, but I wasn't sure how he'd feel about me getting bouquets of flowers from someone else, so I just kept quiet, and eventually it slipped from my mind.

In hindsight I realise this was a mistake – it was like I was lying to him by omission. But at the time I headed home in a really good mood, feeling very lucky for the straightforward and loving relationship I had with Adam, and looking forward to what the rest of the weekend had to offer.

I know, I was an idiot.

Chapter Fourteen

Slowly things began to head back to normal. Well, as normal as things got for Adam and me. With a little distance, the horror of Weegate began to ease and I began to realise my response hadn't been a sign of me somehow falling over the precipice. My limits remained as they were, and Adam – as he had then – continued to respect them. Even the weird feeling that I had somehow disappointed him or let him down by not being able to cope with his head fuckery began to ease. I began to feel on a more even keel emotionally. James moved to the back of my mind, too. It was a relief.

Adam was brilliant through it all – loving, filthy and undoubtedly the reason I was able to regain my equilibrium over time, although I no longer mentally rolled my eyes when he asked me if I knew what my safe word was before we started doing something intense.

The thing was, we hadn't done anything massively intense since that weekend. I couldn't decide if I was relieved or a little disappointed. We'd had sex most nights (barring one late shift when I'd got home too exhausted to move) and our filthy late-night chats continued, but we were definitely talking about D/s more than actually doing it. I don't think it was deliberate on either of our parts, but it was the way things had settled – not least because day-to-day life was as busy as ever, with visits to our families, keeping up with work (me) and building a business (him). But even the most ordinary life experiences can be a little more fun with the addition of some kink – and I decided I should take the initiative to help show him I was ready for another new experience (albeit one less likely to break my brain).

It was his birthday. I know what you're thinking, but this was not going to entail me booking a kink cottage or finding some kind of way to hang from the chandeliers; my plans, for the most part, were pretty sedate. Adam had been working really hard so, a few weeks before, I told him to keep the weekend just after his birthday free so I could take him away somewhere to spoil him. And that's what I did.

After much internet-searching and cross-referencing hotel reviews I found somewhere reasonably priced which looked suitably romantic and ideal for a cosy weekend away. Admittedly, with my sense of direction being a bit ropey and my estimation of travelling time being a little on the optimistic side, it took us seven hours to drive there. We stopped for dinner along the way, but the time in the car – reminiscing over the music I was choosing from his iPod, chatting about everything from the kind of teenagers we'd been through to the last albums we'd bought – reminded me just how much I enjoyed being around Adam. Even when the conversation went silent as the towns and cities gave way to countryside, it was the kind of comfortable silence of two people enjoying each other's company but equally happy with their own thoughts and the views. We checked in late – very late! – and disappeared off to bed quickly, happy to begin exploring the following morning.

After a hearty cooked breakfast, we took the opportunity to go for a walk into the nearby village, getting directions (Adam kept track of them – it was for the best) and then crunching our way down the driveway and paths around the fields. When we got to the village we found it was one tiny shop and a pub/hotel. We nipped into the shop and I bought a pile of newspapers, and then we went into the pub. It felt a bit awkward, as it was only around 11 a.m. or so, but we were hopeful that we might be able to get some tea. Little did we know. The landlady, it appeared, took tea very seriously and soon had us ensconced in the otherwise empty back room with cups and saucers in front of us and a pot big enough for half a dozen.

We sat chatting and warming our hands on the cups as we drank for a little while, until I noticed Adam increasingly looking up at the TV, which was positioned in one corner of the room. I wasn't offended, more intrigued. I knew him well enough by now to know there was something specific going on.

'Do you think they have the sports channels? The second day of the test will be starting soon.'

Before we'd started dating I wouldn't even have known what that meant. Now not only did I know my way around cricketing terminology, but I knew just how much he loved it. He was sheepish, but I just laughed and so we asked. And that's how Adam's romantic birthday weekend of hill walking and generally getting away from it all ended up with us spending six hours of the first day drinking cups of tea from a never-ending pot (it turned out the landlady's late husband had liked cricket – this seemed to make her predisposed to like Adam) while I read the papers from cover to cover and he enjoyed watching the match. As he said with some glee when we began the walk back to the hotel after a large, late lunch (it seemed rude not to eat since we'd nursed our tea for so long), 'England are even ahead. What a brilliant day.'

Of course there had to be some smutty fun in there too.

We got drenched walking back to the hotel so took refuge in the bar area where there was a nice open fire. The drinks were alcoholic this time. I finished mine first, part from nerves and part because I knew I had some organising to do. Adam gestured to ask if I wanted another, but I declined before turning slightly pink – I couldn't help it – and telling him I had a surprise for him and he should give me ten minutes or so and then come back to the room.

The look on his face was a picture. We did a lot of filthy things together, but he really loved it when I planned secret things for him. He raised his pint glass in mock toast. 'This really is the best birthday ever.'

I smiled back at him. 'Ha, don't speak too soon. You don't know what I'm up to yet. See you in ten minutes.'

Then I headed upstairs.

I've never been a fan of outfits. Not even for fancy-dress parties, much less where sex is concerned. It's always made me feel a bit ridiculous, and very self-conscious. It's a long time since I was a schoolgirl, I've never been a beer wench, I'm definitely not cheerleader material, and while I wanted to be Wonder Woman, aged eleven, I'm not inclined to dress like her either. That said, Adam was a fan. He'd told me from the start that he loved underwear, outfits, uniforms and different materials like leather and latex.

I'd mocked him for it. Rolled my eyes at him when I'd seen his eyes linger on my over-the-knee stripey socks. But I knew he was into all this stuff. And it soon became apparent that he genuinely loved the effort, the colour and the fantasy of it all. It wasn't a deal-breaker – it wasn't that he could only enjoy sex that way – and he didn't pressure me to wear things for him, but as I began to realise exactly how much he loved it, it became something I enjoyed doing sometimes to please him and make his eyes light up.

That didn't mean I didn't find the idea a bit silly, not to mention a bit nerve-wracking. The first time I'd dressed up for him, I'd created a little makeshift schoolgirl uniform out of a knee-length grey skirt, white blouse, long socks and an old tie I bought in a charity shop for about 50p. He'd come to visit me and found me on my knees, blindfolded (as much for my benefit as his – I blame the nerves). When he finally took the blindfold off and I got to see how much he adored looking at me in what I considered fancy dress, I became a bit of a convert. It was like he couldn't take his eyes off me and he stared with such hunger and lust that it made me feel a bit more confident, although admittedly still somewhat blushy. He always made me feel good about myself, even when doing degrading things to me, but the way he stared when I tried on a new outfit for the first time gave me goosebumps.

When I wore a corset in front of him for the first time he practically tackled me to the bed and spent an age kissing my breasts as they swelled over the constricting garment. And it wasn't all about the sex outfits. At a friend's wedding I dressed in a demure retro-style fifties dress with a print of tiny cherries on it. At odd moments throughout the day I would catch him staring at me in it, with a look in his eyes that I had come to know and love but which, alas, heralded something we most definitely couldn't do in polite company. When we got back to the hotel we'd booked into overnight we were grabbing at each other, kissing hungrily as soon as we'd closed the door. Of course, he somewhat negated the demureness of the dress by having me undo the halter neck and reveal my breasts before lifting the multi-layered skirt to touch myself for him. But it seemed rude to quibble.

I knew, from the quiet chats we had lying in bed in the dark, that he was a big fan of latex. I had no experience of latex and thus no real opinion either way. But suffice to say, I was a fan of him. And it was his birthday.

I ordered the dress online. It was reasonably well priced and when I tried it on I was surprised not just at how it fitted, accentuating all the right curves but not making me feel self-conscious about the bumpier bits, but at how it felt. It felt lovely against my skin and I found myself stroking it, running my hand along my thigh, enjoying the feeling on my fingertips. It had a zip that ran from the very bottom of the dress – around mid-thigh – right the way up to the neck. Having tested it, I decided that positioning the zipper a little lower, so he could see a hint of cleavage, was the way forward. The zip was incredibly useful as it minimised the inevitable struggle of trying to wrestle yourself into the tight latex. There was still a bit of tussling, though.

I quickly changed; there was a fair amount of arm flailing but I managed to get dressed within the time limit we'd agreed. By the time I heard his card in the door fifteen minutes later – he was clearly making sure I had time to get ready – I'd even stopped heavy breathing at the exertion. I was hoping the flush in my cheeks looked alluring rather than harassed.

When he saw me he actually gasped, which I was hoping was a good sign. I was on my knees, my hands behind my back and crossed at the wrists (it meant I didn't have to worry about nervously twitching my fingers, plus it pushed my breasts out nicely), waiting for him. I still felt shy – I'd deliberately left the light in the room low, although I realised belatedly that I hadn't taken the moonlight from the window into account – but the look in his eyes gave me confidence. Lustful. His whole expression screamed, 'This is amazing, it's like it's my birthday'. And, of course, it was.

He walked over to me and crouched down so he was almost at eye level. His hands reached out and touched the material, stroking up and down my body, then grasping, as if he wanted to get as much of my latex-covered breasts in his hands as possible.

'Oh my fucking God.'

This is not the kind of reaction I am used to getting for my outfit choices. I say this with no sense of self-pity, just the realism of a woman who wears minimal make-up, owns more geeky T-shirts that she does dresses and never learned to wear heels. I smiled up at him. His reaction was exactly what I had hoped for. More, actually. It definitely made the self-consciousness worthwhile.

He leaned down to kiss me, and I arched up to him eagerly. As our tongues moved he continued to run his hands over me. After a long time – not that I was complaining – he stood up in front of me. He started to unbutton his jeans but I reached out and put my hand over his to stop him. He looked down at me with a raised eyebrow. I could tell he was deliberating over whether to grab my wrists and take control or see what I had planned. My throat was a little clogged as I prepared to speak up, but I'd thought about this over and over in my head, running through it.

'Let me,' I whispered.

He returned my smile and, as I started to move, helped me to my feet. As soon as I was upright I wrapped my arms round his neck and started to kiss him eagerly. I pushed my body against him and my tongue into his mouth, controlling the kiss, teasing him and making him groan as his hands found my arse. I smiled as I continued to massage his tongue with mine, shifting us round slightly so that his back was to the bed. I pulled away from him and gently pushed him down onto the mattress, immediately following and crawling up his body, remaining on all fours as I kissed him again. His hands returned to stroking and groping me through the dress.

I wouldn't have described Adam as a switch. By his own admission, he was a big wuss when it came to pain and he didn't like being humiliated or embarrassed. However, from time to time he did love just lying back and enjoying me teasing the life out of him. His tolerance for teasing was actually far higher than mine (and he certainly didn't harrumph if I slowed down as he got close to orgasm as I sometimes did when the tables were turned).

I would kiss him or lick him or suck him, rub his shoulders or scratch between his shoulder blades. It tended to be something I did when I could see he was stressed or tired. He told me it made a nice change to just switch off his brain. He said that he loved the mental challenge of dominating me but it meant he always had to be paying very close attention and planning his next move. This way he felt like he was being spoiled without having to think: he just got to relax instead. It was rare that he craved this, but I could tell when he did and – let's face it – I could relate to enjoying those feelings more than most. I loved fussing over him that way; it was an intimate way for me to show him how much I loved him.

So, when I took hold of his wrists and firmly pulled his hands away from my body, pinning them above his head on the pillow, he didn't complain. He actually smiled eagerly. I reached for the bedside table and took a short length of rope that I'd packed for just this purpose, wrapping his wrists together and tying them to the headboard. It was a fairly crude piece of bondage and one he could have got out of quite easily I'm sure (I didn't have Adam's shibari rope bondage skills – in fact, I'd been rubbish doing knots at Brownies), but he clearly didn't want to wriggle free so I didn't waste too much time worrying about it.

After he was bound I sat up, straddling his waist and feeling his erection pressing against my arse through his jeans. I moved my hips just a little, making him gasp again. I winked at him.

I reached down and slowly unbuttoned his shirt, gently touching and stroking his skin as it came into view. As I reached the last button I pulled the shirt open and dived down to kiss him once more, this time making sure to rub the latex up and down against his bare chest and stomach in a way that made him shiver. I moved from his mouth, kissing down his chin and neck and then round to his ear. I nibbled on his earlobe and whispered, telling him to make himself comfortable because he was going to be here a while. He pushed his pelvis up at these words and let out a low growl – arousal and frustration mixed together, a noise I'd made enough times myself.

I let my lips and tongue explore his shoulder and then moved down his body. I stroked and sucked on his nipples, baring my teeth a little just to remind him of all the times he had bitten mine, making him laugh. I made sure that he still felt the latex on him wherever possible, too, so that by the time my mouth had reached his belly button he was squirming and moaning almost constantly. I loved watching him pull against his bindings as he arched his back. He was starting to look desperate, which is exactly what I wanted. Also, it was rather a novelty for me. I smiled at him. I couldn't help myself. I wondered if this kind of smugness was catching.

I got to the waistband of his jeans and slowly unfastened the buttons. He eagerly lifted his hips so I could pull his trousers down his legs. I also took the opportunity to remove his socks at the same time – they're never a sexy look.

His erection was straining against his boxer shorts. I couldn't resist and moved quickly, giving the material a quick lick, causing his whole body to shudder. I loved that he became so sensitive when teased like this.

I pulled his boxer shorts down and watched as his swollen cock sprang free, looking thicker than usual. It was tempting to put it in my mouth straight away but I had a plan to stick to.

I put my knees either side of his and smiled down at him once again. He actually looked almost sleepy as he stared back. His lips were dry and he kept licking them. If it were me in his position, I might have been begging him to touch me by now. He always did have more self-control. Of course, the difference was I didn't mind if he didn't beg.

I did touch him, but maybe not quite as he hoped. I gently ran my fingernails up his thigh, coming within centimetres of touching his cock and then moving away, scratching up his body and then back down again. The best thing about doing this was watching how his cock would twitch as I got close to it, as if it was involuntarily trying to get me to touch it. It made me wet – well, wetter – as I watched it and the look of concentration on his face as he moaned under his breath.

I smiled. 'You're purring.'

He shook his head. 'Sweetheart, I don't purr. It's a low growl.'

I laughed. 'Oh really? In that case I'll keep going for a bit longer.'

The noise he made then was most definitely a growl.

I loved torturing him like this and kept it up for longer than I had planned, eventually leaning down and kissing his thighs and stomach, but carefully avoiding his cock at all times. I could see how wet his tip was and I was proud of myself for resisting. I'm not sure he felt the same way.

I got up and walked away from the bed. His moan of

disappointment made me chuckle. He was definitely getting desperate.

I walked to the bathroom for a moment and returned with another part of his surprise. I'd brought the bottle of champagne with me from home, but the ice bucket and glasses had been supplied by the hotel at my request. It all felt quite classy and decadent, if you ignored the slutty latex dress and his erection sticking up in the air.

I placed the bucket down on the bedside table and was relieved to find the bottle not too difficult to open. I gradually filled just one of the flutes and took a sip while he watched me, looking amused but a little confused too.

When I brought the glass to my lips for a second time I took more of a mouthful of the champagne. However, instead of swallowing, I held the cold, fizzing liquid in my mouth as I climbed back onto the bed and slipped my lips over his cock.

He cried out as I swirled the champagne round him with my tongue before moving up and down. He was back to muttering profanities at me in which the word 'fuck' featured prominently – it was all quite complimentary in a slightly aggressive way. I made eye contact with him and smiled as the liquid gradually warmed up and lost its fizz. I removed my mouth and swallowed before reaching for another mouthful and repeating the process.

Eventually, as my glass became emptier, I tipped it to his lips so he could have a sip too. I liked my way of drinking it better, though. Not for polite company, admittedly, but it worked for us.

I started to use my hands on his shaft and balls, massaging and teasing as I moved my tongue around him.

I shifted my position so that I was on my knees on the bed with my arse facing him. From this position I knew he'd be able to see up the latex dress. I was bare and – by this point – very wet underneath the dress. I blushed at the thought of his view but I knew he'd love it, even before he told me so and called me his dirty girl.

I quickened my pace and I heard his breath begin to get fast and shallow, which meant only one thing. It was time to stop.

I thought he might go mad from this level of teasing but I wanted to give him one more treat before I finally gave him relief. I moved up the bed and straddled his face so that he was staring straight up at my wetness.

He loved going down on me and one of his favourite positions to do this was for me to ride his face. I know, face-sitting is supposedly the mainstay of dominant women. Not with Adam. He said he didn't really care if this wasn't a particularly dominant way to do it, it got him off. He was never someone concerned by trying to maintain an air of superiority – which explained his stupid naked dances round the bedroom on a Saturday morning while serenading me with whatever song was playing on the radio. He knew that when the dynamic changed I would submit to him without question, and the rest of the time we could just be us.

Of course, he wasn't going to get what he wanted that easily. I kept myself just inches away from his face and slowly rolled up the dress so I could spread my legs a little wider. I reached down and gently stroked my fingers up and down my lips. He loved watching me masturbate; usually I found it a bit embarrassing to do, but in this situation, teasing him in this way, I grinned as my face flushed.

He was able to be much more vocal than I would have been in that situation and started telling me how much he loved watching this and how much it turned him on. I pushed my fingers deep inside myself and moaned as I realised how desperate I was for relief too. I removed my hand and circled his lips, coating them in my wetness. He licked them eagerly and then sucked on my fingers hungrily.

I rubbed myself while he whispered filthy things to me, practically begging me to let him lick me. I held out as long as I could but eventually his offer was just too good to pass up, and I sank down onto his mouth.

Adam's tongue was inside me within a second, pushing in deeper than I thought possible. He strained against the rope as he moved his head. He was desperately trying to taste and lick me, moaning as he did so. He removed his tongue for a second to flick it over my clit before returning to fucking me with it. We were both frantic. As I approached orgasm I lifted for a few seconds to let him take his biggest breath yet and then dropped down again, riding his face as he licked and sucked me, holding onto the headboard for support.

My whole body shook as I came and I lost myself for a moment, coming back to reality, breathing hard and having that awkward post-orgasmic moment of, 'Ooops, have I squashed him?' (surely the occupational hazard of face-sitting). Thankfully I hadn't. I moved off Adam with shaky legs and lay down next to him, finding it hard to look at his face, which was soaking wet with my juices. It didn't help that he was grinning from ear to ear.

I wrapped my arms round him and buried my face in

his neck, which not only felt wonderful for me post-orgasm (I often feel a little clingy in the immediate aftermath but Adam is good with the reassurance), but also meant he was feeling the latex against him once again. I looked down his body to see his toes curling beyond his throbbing cock. Poor boy. I'd have to do something about that in a minute, once I'd recovered.

It took a while, though, and I almost fell asleep in my post-orgasm bliss, until Adam cleared his throat loudly and raised his eyebrows at me as I looked up.

'Something I can help you with?' I smiled at him.

He let out a noise of exasperation and I mocked him a little more before finally relenting and moving down the bed. I sat up and straddled him once again, lowering myself down but deliberately trapping his cock against his stomach. He moaned as I moved my hips, sliding myself up and down his shaft without letting it slip inside. He finally whispered, 'Please', and I relented, lifting slightly and letting him slip inside me.

His groan of relief was so strong that I thought for a moment he had come straightaway. I honestly wouldn't have blamed him – by this point I'd been teasing him for ages. Then he started moving his pelvis, trying to fuck me. I wasn't done being in control just yet, though, so I pinned him to the bed. He stilled. We remained, unmoving, staring at each other, waiting to see what would happen next.

I smiled at him. 'You have so much more self-control than me.'

He nodded. 'Yep. But you're kinder to me than I am to you.'

I nodded and then leaned down to kiss him. 'It's OK, though. It's fun when you're mean.'

He laughed. 'I'll remind you of that next time you're glaring at me.'

Touché. Slowly I reached up and pulled the zip down on my dress, exposing my cleavage further, releasing my breasts. I leaned down and presented them to him, and he began to lick and suck hungrily. I pulled the zip down a little further to give him some more access and he took my nipples in his mouth in turn, flicking his tongue over them. I couldn't resist any more and my hips began to move, up and down, backwards and forwards over his cock. He gasped and moaned into my chest as I fucked him, getting quicker and quicker.

He pulled his head free of my breasts and moaned, 'Please can I come?'

It was the first time he'd ever asked me such a thing (although afterwards he claimed it was because he didn't want to ruin any other plans I had, rather than asking permission per se. I remain unconvinced).

'Of course you can,' I said, more in surprise than anything else. This time I didn't stop moving.

He shouted when he came. If the rest of the hotel didn't know we were in here having sex before then they did now – maybe breakfast in the room tomorrow morning was a plan. I felt his cock twitch and fill me. His orgasm seemed to last for ages before he finally collapsed back, eyes shut, exhausted.

I quickly untied his arms and helped him move them back to his sides. He said they had gone to sleep a bit but would be fine.

I stood up and took off the latex dress, enjoying the cool air on my skin after the warmth of the dress for a few moments before I got back into bed to snuggle up to him. I'd have asked him if he enjoyed his birthday present but he was already fast asleep – I didn't take offence and considered it a sign things had gone quite well. I mocked him for it when he roused a little later – but then he asked for a glass of champagne and we started all over again.

We did end up having breakfast in the room the next morning. It just seemed less embarrassing somehow. Plus it meant we didn't need to get dressed.

Chapter Fifteen

Not telling Adam when James sent me flowers was one thing. When he turned up at my office suddenly, it felt like something I might have to bring up, no matter how awkward it felt.

It was a week or two after Adam's birthday. I'd had a couple of manic weeks at work, but the big redesign we were all working on was coming to an end and I was looking forward to getting through the afternoon and heading out for celebratory drinks later.

I was dashing out to buy a sandwich to see me through the afternoon when I, almost literally, bumped into James. My first thought was one of suspicion. His office was over the other side of the city, so the chances that he was just walking past in the middle of the day were pretty slim. He raised his hand to wave hi and, while I wanted to pretend I hadn't seen him, I figured he'd just follow me if I tried to dash off.

'Hello.' He smiled.

'Hi.' I didn't. This felt incredibly awkward. I'm rubbish at reading the signs of what's going on in these situations at the best of times. My experiences with James had proved that I found him more difficult to read than anyone else. I could do without this. I didn't say anything else.

'Are you heading out for lunch?'

I swallowed down my irritation. It was 1.10 p.m. on a Friday afternoon. The chances were high. 'No. I'm going out on a job.'

He looked at me for a long moment. 'Can I buy you a sandwich before you go out?'

We both knew I was lying about the job. And he clearly had something he wanted to talk about. I was curious, proof of my masochistic tendencies, if more were needed. Maybe clearing the air was a good idea. I sighed and began walking down the street as he began following me.

'I'll buy my own sandwich.'

By the time we'd ordered our sandwiches I was wondering why on earth I'd thought this was a good idea. It was hideously awkward. I kept sneaking looks at James's face when he wasn't looking. He looked more unsettled than I'd ever known him to be. In the end, as was so often the case, I cracked first. 'What's up? Are you OK?'

He took a sip of his drink and nodded slowly. 'Yeah, I'm fine. Good.'

A long pause. This was going brilliantly, not least because I wasn't actually sure I cared whether he was alright.

'I was at a meeting nearby so I thought I'd come and hang around to see if you were about so we could catch up.'

So many sarcastic comments flitted through my mind. I tried to ignore them for something safer. 'You should have rung.'

He smiled wryly. He knew me too well. He knew what I was thinking. 'I did consider it, but you either have a new mobile number or have been ignoring my messages. I thought about ringing your office but I was hoping the element of surprise might work in my favour.'

I smiled in spite of myself; it was a rueful smile. It felt weird that someone I had felt such a connection to, felt so in love with, could be sitting opposite me like a stranger. Worse than a stranger – an unwelcome acquaintance. 'And how's that gone for you?'

He laughed, an echo of previous times. 'Not brilliantly. I don't think this is the most happy you've ever been to see me.'

His mouth was smiling but his eyes were sombre. I couldn't even summon up a quirk of my lips. My patience levels were low and I'd tired of the game. It was like picking at a scab. 'Why are you really here, James?'

His voice was hesitant. 'To ask you out for dinner.'

It was ironic to think there was a time I'd have felt excited at him doing that. Not now. I wanted to kick him in the shins for hurting me so badly. I took a long look at him. He looked a bit tired, slightly defeated. It was like he knew what my answer would be before I gave it.

'I can't.' Shit, this was what had worried me when I wrote that email. Ambiguity is why this is so difficult. 'I don't want to,' I clarified. Bit harsh? Maybe. I tried to temper it. 'I just don't think it's a good idea. I'm in a new relationship now, and I'm happy. Going to dinner, even innocently –' (I thought the caveat was important, I still had no bloody clue exactly what he was thinking) '– would feel wrong. In fact, this feels wrong.'

He looked hurt. I felt a pang of guilt at hurting him, until he spoke at least. 'Look, it doesn't matter that you're seeing Thomas still. I've tried to forget you too. I can't. I wondered if you'd like to try again.' He smiled slightly. 'Or try properly really, because we never really did.'

I felt such a surge of rage I didn't even know where to begin. 'No, we never really did. That was your choice. And you told me you loved me then, but then buggered off anyway. I don't want to try anything with you.'

He opened his mouth to reply but I cut him short before he could. 'And it's nothing to do with Tom. I've met someone else. We're living together, we're happy, we have a life together.'

He looked confused, sheepish, surprised that I might have found someone else. It made me want to pour his coffee in his lap. 'But I loved you. I love you,' he replied.

They were words I'd have given so much to hear when I needed them most but now that's all they were – hollow words. Suddenly I was tired.

'James, you don't love me. I'm sorry if you're hurting but this isn't love. Remember when you said you loved me and that's why you found it so difficult to inflict pain on me and had to step back from dominating me?'

He nodded.

'Well, don't you think if you'd loved me then you'd have missed just seeing me without any D/s, or any sex at all?'

He interrupted then, but it was a bit half-hearted, the protestation of a small boy who's been caught out. 'I did miss you. I do.'

I shook my head. 'If you'd missed me you wouldn't have been able to stay away. But you did. And it's fine, I'm not offended really. You probably did me a favour. We weren't going to work long term. I needed the reassurance, someone who I knew where I was with. No second-guessing, no wondering.'

His question was part curiosity, part wistfulness. 'Have you got that now?'

I didn't see the point in answering, felt no need to justify my relationship with Adam to him. I didn't want to talk about something so special with him when it wasn't his business. But I knew in my heart that the answer to his question was a definite yes.

We finished lunch quickly, with the bare minimum of awkward small talk, but I felt relieved that it was done. He said he'd keep in touch as friends but we both knew, as he kissed me on the cheek, that he wasn't going to. And I was OK with that.

By the time I walked back to the office for the afternoon, I had the beginnings of a headache forming across the bridge of my nose. I'm not great with confrontation, and while I knew that I'd done the right thing, I hated the fact I might have hurt his feelings, even while I felt a burning annoyance that he seemed to think he could slope back into my life after months of silence.

I also knew I'd have to tell Adam that we'd met. I didn't know how he'd react, and while things had settled down since our trip to York, and his business was going well, I didn't want to do anything that made him feel unsure about my feelings for him. I also didn't want to make it seem like James was still a factor in my life – it was quite awkward, given that we'd talked a lot about my feelings for James early on, back when I'd not even considered a relationship with Adam as a possibility.

It was all so bloody complicated.

Of course, when we finally got to the pub for my evening work do, it didn't help when Mark jokingly told Adam off for showing up the blokes in the office by sending ostentatious bouquets of flowers.

Adam's eyes flickered over to me. I knew I looked stricken and a bit guilty, but what could I say at that point? He smiled at Mark and said, 'Sorry, mate', and the conversation moved on, but I knew it would come up later. He wasn't daft, and he wasn't someone who'd just let that pass without asking about it, even though he knew that it was probably all innocent.

Except now it didn't feel innocent. It felt like an accidental betrayal. And paired with having to tell him about my impromptu lunch with James earlier that day, it was suddenly looking like we'd have to have a potentially hideous conversation.

Shit.

We got a lift back with Shona, who'd got the weekend shift and so hadn't been drinking. We all chatted easily enough in the car about the traffic, the weather, all those random things that fill the silence. But then we were home and I had a ball of nerves in the pit of my stomach.

To his credit, he didn't let me stew about it.

I started taking my coat off and he moved into the kitchen to switch the kettle on, as much for something to do, I think, as anything else.

'So what's the deal with the flowers?' He had his back to me, so I couldn't tell how casual and laid-back he actually was, but his tone was calm. I took a deep breath.

'James sent them.'

He put the tin holding the teabags back into the cupboard with more force than strictly necessary. 'I don't remember you bringing them home. When was this?'

I hesitated. 'A month or two ago now. The night I went out for cocktails with Charlotte. I gave them to her, I didn't want them.'

He turned to look at me, his eyes watchful, wary in a way that made me feel rotten. 'Why didn't you tell me?'

So many possible answers. I decided to keep it simple. 'It didn't seem important. It felt inappropriate to bring them home, so I gave them to Charlotte instead. I just didn't think to mention it.'

'Inappropriate'? How had this got so stupidly formal?

'Charlie took them?'

I nodded.

'And did she know who they were from?'

I nodded again, albeit slightly confused. Why did that matter? His face definitely said that it did.

'So why tell her and not tell me?'

I shrugged my shoulders. 'It honestly didn't seem important. We didn't have a massive conversation about them, I just told her when I handed them over.' I thought it best to leave out that I'd deliberately not mentioned it until she was getting into her cab so she didn't get a chance to question me about it further.

He scanned my face looking for more. It made me nervous. Times like this, him knowing me so well, didn't work in my favour.

'So why did he send you flowers?'

I sighed. There was no way not to have this conversation now. 'He asked me out.' I tried to smile, but he didn't return it. 'Obviously I said no.'

His arms were now crossed against his chest. He looked harsh but also hurt. I wanted to make it better but had no bloody clue how to, just a certain knowledge he wasn't going to like what I said next, although it had to be said.

'I saw him today and told him about you. How happy we are, how I'm not interested in anything with him any more.'

'You saw him? Where?'

'He came to my office.' I swallowed before continuing. 'We went for lunch.'

His voice was suddenly brusque. 'You went on a lunch date with him?'

The cold anger in his voice suddenly made me furious. 'Of course I didn't go on a bloody lunch date with him. He was lurking outside my office waiting to invite me for lunch. I decided it was best to go and just tell him I wasn't interested in person to get it over with.'

'Really?' He didn't sound convinced.

'Really.'

'And were you going to tell me you'd met him for lunch?'

I could feel my voice getting more shrill as I got angry, but I couldn't stop myself. 'Of course I was.'

His laugh was bitter. 'How am I supposed to believe that when you didn't even tell me he'd got back in touch?'

I was starting to panic. We didn't really have rows in our house when I was growing up and a hangover of that upbringing was that I hated this kind of confrontation. If I'm honest, I was crap at coping with it. I had no idea what to say, hated the fact I'd upset him and yet felt a burning sense of injustice and a rising sense of anxiety. I couldn't cock this up now.

'Don't be like that, I didn't think about it. It wasn't important. It isn't important. James has no bearing on my life now, certainly no bearing on us.'

Adam's faced was screwed up with an emotion I couldn't quite understand, and his tone made me flinch. 'I think he has quite a big bearing on us. Not least because when we started seeing each other you weren't anywhere near being over him. You'd stepped back for self-preservation purposes when he went quiet, but it was obvious you still liked him. If nothing else, you told me so.'

I couldn't speak for a moment. He was jealous. It felt odd – it was daft that he knew me so well, could read my emotions better than anyone I'd met and yet could be so stupidly blind.

'That was ages ago, you bloody idiot. Do you think I'd have started a relationship with you, much less moved in with you and started building a life together if I secretly hoped I could get back together with another man?'

Adam's mouth dropped open at the anger in my tone, but there wasn't time for him to interrupt quite yet.

'I love you, you moron. You're my person. When I wake up in the morning and see your head resting on the pillow next to me, everything feels right with the world. When something good happens, or something bad, my first instinct is to share it with you. I've never been as honest, spoken as frankly, with anyone as I have with you. You make me laugh.' My voice softened. 'I wonder what our babies might look like, whether they'd have your hair or my eyes. I think about

286

what it'll be like to get old with you, what we'll do when my knees get so creaky that if I kneel in front of you you'll have to help me up afterwards. When I think about my life I can't imagine you not being in it now. You aren't some kind of back-up in case I can't find someone better. You are the best. You're the one. I love you, you stupid arse.'

I turned round to look out the window, suddenly incredibly self-conscious and a bit tearful. I stared at the road outside, trying to pull myself together for whatever happened next.

Suddenly his arms were sliding round me from behind, his body warm and comforting and solid behind me. With every fibre of my being I wanted to lean back, to lean into him and yield, but I stayed upright. Suspicious. Unsure.

He rested his chin on my shoulder. I could see his reflection in the window and while he wasn't smiling he didn't look angry any more. He sighed quietly and his breath against my neck made me shiver.

'I'm sorry. I know I'm an idiot. I was just surprised that you hadn't told me. It's not like you.'

I turned round and opened my mouth to reply, but he put his fingers against my lips.

'I know. I know you didn't want to upset me. I bet they were some kind of gold-plated bouquet and you were worried I'd feel bad about that too, especially if it was not long after I was made redundant.' I smiled, in spite of myself. 'It was just a shock to hear he was back in your life and you were giving him the time of day.'

I bit my lip. 'Adam, it wasn't like that. He's not back. He knows I'm not interested.'

He pressed a kiss to my forehead. It was a tiny gesture,

one he had done hundreds of times before, but the sheer relief that he had done it again almost made my knees buckle.

'I know it wasn't like that, sweetheart. And I know you think I'm mental. But when we met you were still consumed by him, even though he had treated you so shabbily and I knew you deserved better. The fact that he came back to try again is pretty much my worst nightmare.'

I sighed. 'But I'm not going anywhere.'

He smiled. 'I know, and that's amazing. But I didn't know that to start with, did I?'

I shook my head somewhat sheepishly. 'No. I suppose not.'

'The thing is, I love you too. I don't say it as much as you do, although I am getting better on that front, but I try and show you every day,' he waggled his eyebrows, 'and not even just in sexy ways.' I rolled my eyes. 'I can't imagine my life without you in it either. It'd be quite boring. Tidier, probably. But if we broke up my parents would be very disappointed. They'd given up on me ever finding anyone to put up with me.'

I pulled a face at him. 'Wow, so you're settling with me then as the only woman who'll put up with your ways?'

He nipped my bottom lip in playful warning, and grinned. 'It's not that you're the only woman who'll put up with me. It's that you're the only woman who can keep up with me.'

I think my face must have fallen a little, because suddenly he was pressing kisses to my face again.

'No, no, no, not just that. Don't get me wrong, I love the sex we have, but I think what makes it so intense and fun is our emotional as well as physical connection. I know partly that connection comes from us being able to talk to each other about pretty much anything,' he touched my cheek, 'even if sometimes it makes you blush.'

My lips quirked.

'I love you, Soph. The real thing. The spending our lives together, getting through the ups and downs, looking after each other, loving each other whole caboodle.'

I couldn't hide the frustration in my voice. 'Well, why are we arguing then?'

He kissed me again. 'Because I get perturbed when you're not characteristically open and honest with me.'

I swallowed hard. 'I know, and I'm sorry. I was going to tell you.'

Adam smiled. 'I know you were. I believe you.' He pressed his mouth to mine, and I opened my mouth, eager for a proper (or, OK, improper) kiss. Before I got the chance, though, he'd broken away again. 'Oh and for the record, "I love you, you stupid arse"? Very smooth.'

I kicked him in the shin with my bare foot and he kissed me.

Chapter Sixteen

I'm not good with rows, but there was something about my post-pub chat with Adam that cleared the air like a summer storm. Was I glad it had happened so dramatically? No, and there were a good few weeks afterwards where I felt the urge to reassure him of how much I loved him – and, if I'm honest, needed similar reassurance that he no longer felt upset at me. But all it did, weirdly but happily, was make us stronger, not just as an ordinary couple but in D/s terms.

One of the things that I found most interesting about submitting to Adam was that his type of domination was so different to that I had experienced before. There were some similarities in how the people I had played with before had controlled me, but the most notable thing was that there was a lot of pain involved. That didn't bother me, in fact quite the opposite – my masochistic tendencies and enjoyment of the endorphin rush meant it felt pretty amazing – but Adam's style was different. He was far from being a sadist. I knew he'd had submissive partners before that were really into pain – it's not an unusual trait to find in a sub, after all – but he seemed to get off on seeing a woman *enjoy* the pain, rather than purely from inflicting it. He was a complex man, nothing if not surprising.

Sometimes, though, even I was astonished at how and

where we managed to discover kink. One weekend we were in a large sports store so Adam, who had begun cycling to both get fit and save petrol money, could buy some new lights for his bike.

I was wide-eyed at the huge warehouse-like shop. I like swimming and go to the gym, but otherwise I haven't played sport since my days in a netball skirt at secondary school. And certainly things have changed on the shopping front since then. We had just walked past the wetsuit aisle when we got to the equestrian goods.

I may have enjoyed our recent forays into pet play but becoming a 'pony girl' didn't really interest me – or Adam, as far as I knew. However, something clearly put a spring in his step; his pace quickened and I hurried after him. He had a grin on his face that could only mean he'd seen something he found exciting – he really was like a big kid at times; it was just as well I found it – and him – endearing.

I followed his gaze and noticed a large selection of riding crops. Adam had recently broken his crop mid-session – thankfully not as painful as it sounded – and I'd had to bite my lip to stop myself laughing at his forlorn look as he hid the two pieces in the rubbish. It seemed he wanted to pick up a replacement.

Just as we did at the pet shop, we stood in that run-of-the-mill shop surrounded by weekend bargain hunters, and in hushed tones discussed purchasing what seemed like an ordinary item for kink purposes. I'd like to say that I was blushing less this time round, but I really wasn't. It was only my eye for a bargain that stopped me fleeing back to admire the snorkelling gear. What surprised us both was that not only were the crops identical to the ones we had seen online and in sex shops – obviously some supplier had two very different types of customer – but they were about a quarter of the price. You accept that you generally have to pay over the odds for sex toys and equipment, for well-made stuff it's just a kink tax that has to be endured. However, this was like finding the ultimate sex toy discount and we selected a lovely looking crop that had a price tag of something ridiculous like £4.

My ears were hot by the time he picked it up off the rack but I was actually almost as excited as him at such a bargain. Well, that and also the fact that this was a pretty good sign we were going to head home for an afternoon of lovely, endorphin-heavy fun.

We were about to walk away when Adam stopped, eyes wide. I wasn't sure that this was a good sign, especially when I saw what he was looking at. I couldn't swallow my gasp. The sign said 'dressage whip' and it was about 30 inches in length, not dissimilar to the crop in many ways but much longer and thinner. About three quarters of the way up the shaft the strong but flexible core seemed to come to an end but the material carried on, hanging limply from the end like a thick shoelace.

I knew with certainty that it would hurt. A lot. I stared at it, wondering what the marks would look like, how long they would last. It was in his hands in a moment and as he flexed it, trying the weight, his eyes narrowing as he thought about how it would swing, I won't deny that it fascinated me too. Not that I necessarily wanted him to buy it. But, of course, he did – it was a new toy for him to play with. I would have called his excitable face at his second bargain of the day 'cute' – if I didn't know how he planned to play with the toy when we got home.

Almost as soon as we got back to our flat, he was fishing around in one of his many well-organised boxes of toys. It didn't take him long to find his flogger, which had a weighty black leather handle with many thick, almost suede-like tails coming from the end. It was something that he could stroke over my body, causing me to break out in goosebumps, or strike heavy blows and bring up welts with. In spite of that, OK *because of that*, I loved it.

The flogger, crop and whip were laid out in the living room and I almost dared to hope he was just obsessively organising his collection rather than planning something. He wouldn't, couldn't, use all three in one go, could he? Ah, who was I kidding with my wide-eyed optimism?

Once he'd laid them out as he wanted, he noticed me watching and smiled. He grabbed hold of me and started to kiss me, his arms snaking around my back, pulling me close. I melted into him, forgetting the slightly worrying pile on the coffee table and just focusing on his embrace.

His hands didn't stay where they were for long. At first he was stroking my back and then he grabbed my top and pulled it up, breaking our kiss for just a moment as he lifted it over my head.

Next my bra was unfastened and within moments my jeans and knickers were round my ankles. We shared a laugh as we continued to kiss – he really had become quite adept at making me naked very quickly.

He stood back so I could shed my now-useless clothing, and once again he was fully dressed and I didn't have a stitch on. He made me stand with my legs shoulder-width apart and my hands behind my head, fingers interlocked. He made me wait, and I enjoyed the building nerves as I watched him, trying to figure out what I needed to prepare myself for. Then he picked up the flogger, and I bit back a smile, knowing he was saving his new toys in the same way he saved his roast potatoes during Sunday lunch, because they were his favourite bit and thus should – in his world – be eaten last.

He stroked the tails of the flogger up and down my body, making my breasts tingle and my nipples harden. He then stood behind me and did the same to my back and legs, making me struggle not to shake a little with nerves.

But then he stopped stroking and started swinging. Not hard at first, in fact it was barely noticeable, but as the minutes passed the flogger was definitely moving further away from my body and being swung back harder onto it. It still felt nice, but gradually the strikes became more and more intense. He was warming me up. It was working.

Eventually I was feeling real impact on my arse and thighs. It still wasn't what I'd call painful but as he swung his arm and the strands of the flogger hit me together it felt like a solid thud rather than a number of different tails stinging me.

The blows got harder and harder, until I was wincing with the impact every time he hit my arse. He then started to move round my body, striking all round my legs, stomach and breasts as I grimaced. He varied from swinging his arm as though he was wielding a tennis racquet to turning his wrist in circles so that he was suddenly hitting me with just the tips of the suede tails rather than the full length. Each variation was a different sensation to experience and endure.

I wasn't sure he'd ever spent so long using the flogger on me before, but I could tell he was monitoring me closely, not just to see if I was OK but to understand what reactions he was getting when he changed where and how he hit me. That knowledge slowed the nerves cramping my stomach.

He even swung down and hit the tops of my feet, which resulted in a cry of surprise from me. That was nothing compared to the cry I let out when he swished between my legs and caught my clit.

By the time he stopped, it seemed that there wasn't a part of my body that hadn't felt the thud or sting of the flogger. The intensity of the pain hadn't been hard to handle but the length of time he had spent flicking me with the suede fronds made it feel like an endurance test.

The flogger was returned to the table and he reached straight for the dressage whip. I knew before he swished it through the air that this was going to be a different kind of pain. As before, he started with my arse. A couple of soft taps, and then came that swishing noise followed by a sting across my cheeks that made me grit my teeth. Another then another in quick succession before a pause. He knelt down and checked my arse.

'Oh my word, you should see this. Instant thin lines. I think you're going to have some welts.' The wonder in his voice made me feel affection and a weird kind of pride at how pleased he sounded. He may not have been a sadist but he did love to see the marks. Not that I could say anything about that: I was incapable of stopping my fingers from running along my body when bruises blossomed in the days after he hurt me. They were a colourful illustration of the fun we'd had.

No fun yet, though. There was no other way to describe it – the whip hurt like hell. I couldn't help but flinch when I saw him swing and heard the noise as it moved through the air. Where my skin had gone red from the flogger, the thin lines of the whip were even more noticeable. When he whipped my breasts I bit my lip and when he whipped my feet I almost kicked him.

This was definitely the most challenging pain he had put me through and certainly the most pain I had experienced in a long time. Slightly hysterically, I wondered to myself if it was possible my tolerance for it had lowered. It hurt so much. Had it hurt this much before? Had I just forgotten? Eroticised it? How could I cope with this? When would it stop? Would I be able to last?

In a rarity for Adam, he wasn't doing anything else to me while the whipping took place. There was no sense of humiliation or degradation, nothing else for my brain to focus on, challenge or rail against. It was just pain. Harsh, jagged, relentless pain. And, forgive me for stating the bleeding obvious, it hurt. So, so much.

Adam was watching me closely, but now it was less to do with experimentation and more about him checking up on me. That calmed my panicky inner monologue a little. I knew I could trust him, knew he would look after me. I knew I could take more but I could sense a little reticence and concern in him.

He put the whip aside and reached for the crop. OK, maybe the perceived concern was hysterical optimism on my part.

A third implement meant having to try to get used to a whole different intensity and type of pain once again. It stung, especially against the already-lumpy lines left by the whip and the reddened areas of skin courtesy of the flogger. The pain was sharp and direct on a relatively small area, and he swung hard from the start.

He cropped me all over quickly – arse, thighs, stomach, breasts. I didn't know where the next strike would hit and I was starting to find it very challenging, struggling to breathe, to focus on processing the pain. He kept going, further than he ever had before, striking my nipples and then, when I tried to protect myself, hitting my arms until I moved them out of the way and put them back on my head.

My head was swimming and my eyes began to water. The pain was breaking me down but at that point I wanted it, was yearning for the cathartic release. That didn't stop me flinching or gritting my teeth, though. I knew if he kept this up I was going to burst into tears.

Then he stopped. He was in front of my face in an instant. Stroking my hair and kissing my forehead. It was lovely but it felt odd. It was almost like orgasm denial to me at that point – I could take more and I wanted to.

'Please.' I whispered, brokenly. Desperately.

'What do you want, sweetheart?' His voice was tender, tinged with genuine concern.

'You don't have to stop. Please don't stop. I want you to make me cry.'

He touched his forehead to mine. Closed his eyes. After a deep breath he moved back, his gaze searching. 'Are you sure?'

I swallowed and nodded. 'Yes.' I blushed a little. 'Please.'

I'm not sure I'd seen conflict in his face before. He'd always seemed so sure of everything. He put his hands round my throat on a regular basis, but making me cry in pain was one of the few things he hadn't experienced. He'd made my eyes water before, but he had never made me sob, never made me properly weep with pain. I could tell he wasn't sure whether to push me, whether I could cope. But this time I knew. I trusted him, truly trusted him, and I knew.

He'd brought me so close. I wanted to feel tears stream down my face, yearned for the release of my body being racked with sobs, the catharsis of the pain.

For a long moment we looked at each other. Despite my glistening eyes I was smiling. 'Trust me.'

He didn't speak for long seconds. Slowly his mouth curved and he smiled back. 'I trust you.'

He took a deep breath and began again, making sure to hit me at least as hard as he had before. To start with he moved around my body as he had previously, making me guess where the next strike would hit, even hitting between my legs a few more times.

Then he began to focus. The crop struck my breast and I winced. He did it again. And again. He began to strike me harder; he swung his arm back further, I was struggling and I felt the lump in my throat rise. Again and again and again he hit me and all I kept thinking was, 'Please don't stop'.

Then it happened. My mouth had been tightly shut, my lips pressed together as I endured the pain, but one final blow made me open them and cry out. It was the release I had been waiting for. My knees buckled and I collapsed on the floor, tears flowing freely and my body shaking as I began to sob.

He was there in an instant. Crouching with me, arms holding me tight, whispering words of love. I gasped, 'Thank you', over and over again, trying to reassure him that I was OK and that he had done what I wanted, what I had craved, what in that moment I had needed more than anything else.

As I clung to him I felt his erection pressing against me and smiled through the tears, even though I was in no position to do anything about it just yet. Soon, though.

Eventually he picked me up off the floor and took me to bed, lying down with me and making sure everything was really OK. In this instance I think it was as much to reassure himself as it was to reassure me.

As I came back to myself and we continued to cuddle we discussed what had happened, the way we usually did when we'd tried something new. But this time I was asking him how he felt about pushing himself as much as he was asking me how I had enjoyed it.

Softly, we talked. I was exhausted, like I had been broken down and rebuilt, and as he brushed my hair off my shoulders, I told him how much I had enjoyed it, enjoyed being challenged. He kissed me softly on the shoulder, and I turned his head and kissed him deeply on the mouth instead.

As we began moving against each other and he slipped inside me, he broke the kiss and stilled.

For a moment I was worried something was wrong, the expression on his face was so earnest. 'What is it?'

Then he broke into a smile, the wide smile of my Adam, the smile that can be brought about by everything from a toe-curling blow job to a slice of carrot cake to finding a repeat of *Man v. Food* on TV.

His voice was filled with wonder. 'You're so fucking wet.'

I stuck my tongue out at him. 'It's ungentlemanly for you to say so.'

He laughed out loud and kissed my nose. 'You think it's ungentlemanly for me to point that out, but you're OK with me whipping, flogging and cropping you until you cry?'

I looked at him with mock-seriousness. 'That's correct. What's your point?'

His tone was properly serious, though, and still filled with wonder. 'It's incredible. You're incredible. I've never hit anyone until they cried with the pain before. When you started sobbing it was like a wave rushed through you. The release was almost like an orgasm. It was amazing. So sexy to watch. It felt,' he broke off to pull a face, but then continued, 'it sounds lame, but it felt such a privilege to be the one who could break you that way.' He looked sheepish. 'I sound like a pretentious prick.'

I laughed. 'I think it's fair to say most pretentious pricks lack the self-awareness to know that's what they actually are. You're alright.'

He smiled back at me and, in unspoken mutual agreement, we began to move our hips. 'Thank you.'

I grinned and gasped as he grabbed my arse, his fingertips pressing against a plethora of bruises and welts. 'You're welcome. And thank you.'

He kissed my nose. 'You're welcome. And thank you.'

We kept fucking and eventually we stopped thanking each other. It took a while, though. We're nothing if not polite.

Except, you know, when we aren't.

Chapter Seventeen

It might sound a bit strange to say it, but after the catharsis of that afternoon, my life with Adam fell back into its
regular rhythm. Any remaining fears about being pushed
too far had gone, while the conversation about James a
few weeks before seemed to have brought about a kind of
peace born of the fact we both knew better than ever
where we stood. Life was busy and the months passed,
with Adam getting a flurry of new clients for his business
while I took on more freelance work than ever before.
Our weekends were a mixture of the usual social stuff –
families, friends, trips to the cinema – and working in
companionable silence on laptops, stopping only for tea
or occasional moments of friskiness.

It sounds a bit daft to say it, but it remained a novelty
to have a boyfriend whom my parents loved, with whom
I could spend four hours in a pub arguing about the top-
ten film sequels ever made (and whether *The Empire Strikes
Back* still counts as one following the *Star Wars* prequels)
and who didn't get annoyed when I worked weekends or
late nights because he knew how much my job meant to
me. The fact that not only was he the filthiest man I had
ever met but he also took work as seriously as me, and
wanted kids and a home one day, was, frankly, the icing on
the kinky cake.

The sexual side of our relationship didn't slow, but it certainly settled within our wider life together. There was still plenty of stuff that felt intense and challenging, but there was a lot more straightforward sex too – albeit with occasional nipple pinching or a stray spanking here or there.

One particular Saturday we weren't doing anything intense, though. It was early evening, and Adam and I were curled up on the sofa with freshly poured glasses of red wine to toast him completing his first set of accounts for his new copywriting consultancy (the most difficult part of which was, ironically, getting the paperwork from his bank in the first place).

We'd talked about buying somewhere together, mostly pie-in-the-sky stuff, although the rent on our current flat gave us enough leftover money each month to put some aside. With his business doing so well and my freelance work taking off, our savings were looking healthy and we were trying to work out if we were in a position yet to consider making a move. The completion of his accounts was another piece in the jigsaw.

We were discussing the relative merits of waiting for a little while (not least so we could afford to buy some furniture), when my phone pinged.

Initially I ignored it, as we were alternating between waxing lyrical about what our house would be like and coming up with ideas for new clients for Adam's business – ex-colleagues we could tap up for freelance and consultancy work. I hadn't known him to be happier on the work front – he was motivated, enjoying the creativity and the freedom of being his own boss. The Adam who had been so bored with his job before his redundancy, and so negative in its immediate aftermath, was long gone. It was lovely to hear his enthusiasm, and I was enjoying coming up with my own ideas to help him with his venture. The fact that, one day – mortgage lenders allowing – it could enable us to have our own home too was just a bonus.

We were bickering good-naturedly about where my collection of china dragons (don't judge, I collect them) would go when my phone pinged again. One message on a weekend when I wasn't on call for work was easily ignored. Two in quick succession was more of a sign that something was going on. He looked at me, and then nodded to the phone.

'Go on, it's OK. You should check your messages.'

I grabbed my phone and read them. They were both from Thomas.

> Charlotte has ended things
> between us. We're through.

Followed immediately afterwards by:

> Although apparently we
> weren't ever actually together.
> Stupid me. Fancy a beer?

I passed my phone to Adam and he scanned the messages.

'That doesn't sound good. Do you want to ring him?'

I gave him an impulsive hug. Adam's laid-back nature was one of the things I loved most about him, but never more so than then, when the needs of a friend, one who was effectively an ex, had gate-crashed our evening. Not only did he not have a problem with it, but he knew that I would want to check on Tom. In spite of the sexual side of our friendship ceasing long ago, Tom remained one of my best friends – and it took a laid-back boyfriend to be fine with that. That Adam felt secure enough in my love for him to be that relaxed was something I was very grateful for.

'Do you mind?' I gestured to the wine glasses. 'Rain check on this?'

He kissed the top of my forehead. 'It's OK, sweetheart. I can pick your brain for business ideas whenever. Go ring him.' He leaned over to get his own phone. 'I'll text Charlie and see how she's doing.'

Which is how our quiet night in ended up with us in two different bars getting drunk with other people.

By the time I arrived at the bar, Thomas had already clearly had a couple. He also looked more miserable than I had ever seen him.

'Hey you.'

He looked up and waved in half-hearted welcome, before turning his attention back to his drink.

'I'm going to get a beer. Do you want another?' I asked, not sure it was a good idea but not wanting to seem rude. He nodded.

When I got back to the table he was fiddling with his phone.

'I thought I'd text her. But I don't know what to say.'

He looked a bit broken and, to be honest, I wasn't entirely sure what to say either. Let's face it, 'Are you OK?' was out, because he clearly wasn't.

'Do you think texting will help?'

He shook his head dolefully. 'To be honest I don't know there's anything more I can say to her. I think we're done.' His face flashed with grief, as if hearing the words out loud, even from his own mouth, was too much to bear. 'Fuck, I think we're done.'

It seemed surreal. Bearing in mind how happy Charlotte had been when we'd gone out, I couldn't understand what had happened to cause such a change. So I asked.

'What happened?'

He didn't speak for a long time. So long that I wondered if he'd actually heard me. Finally, he replied.

'I told her I loved her. Twice.' He smile was thin-lipped. 'I think it's fair to say she doesn't feel the same way.'

Shit.

'She broke things off? Because of that?'

He nodded. 'The first time I said it, it kind of slipped out. We were lying in bed and she was curled into my arm and I said it.' Something in my expression must have given me away. 'No, don't look like that, it wasn't a post-sex thing. We were just cuddling. It was really nice. Cosy. When I said it, she stiffened a bit, but I thought I'd better just say it properly – I'd spent ages thinking it and having to be careful that I didn't blurt it out. So I told her. I told her I loved her, that I wanted us to be in a proper relationship together.' His voice got quiet. 'That was when she moved away.

'She told me that she didn't want anything serious. She never had. That this was all about having fun sexual experiences with people she liked and trusted. She was quite upset about it, but she also seemed a bit angry at me telling her I had these feelings when we'd always said what we had was casual. I told her that it was fine, we could go back to being friends with benefits, that would be enough. But she said she now knew it wouldn't be enough for me, that I deserved better and that we should end things properly. A clean break.'

I honestly didn't know what to say to make him feel better. In fact, worse than that, I knew there was nothing I could say, no combination of words that could help.

'I'm so sorry, Tom.'

He smiled wanly. 'I know. I'm hoping she'll change her mind, but I'm not optimistic. I'm so stupid for telling her.'

I put my hand across the table to squeeze his. 'You can't help how you feel.'

He shook his head. 'I know, but I'm now going to have to stop feeling it. I just don't understand. A proper relationship was the next step. We had so much fun, we did so much stuff together – munches, parties, threesomes. The sex was literally the best I've ever known.'

I burst out laughing and he looked sheepish.

'I'm sorry, Soph, I didn't mean it like that.' I raised an eyebrow. 'You don't count really.'

I laughed again. 'It's just as well I know what you mean and have a sense of humour or you'd be in so much trouble.'

He looked discomfited but continued doggedly. 'I just think that sexual compatibility, that mutual open-mindedness, would be a great basis for a relationship.'

I nodded. 'Definitely.'

'But it's not enough.'

'No.'

We finished our beers in silence.

*

Adam got home a little after me – I'd poured Tom into a taxi, while Adam (ever the gentleman) had instead seen Charlotte to her front door. I'd picked up my glass of wine and resumed my place on the sofa as soon as I got home, half watching the news channel as someone reviewed the next day's front pages and half letting my mind wander, thinking about how rotten Tom felt and how lucky I'd been in meeting Adam. My fury at the cack-handed matchmaking that had got us in the same room was a distant memory.

He sank down on the sofa next to me and leaned in for a kiss.

'Hey you.'

I smiled and pulled him into a hug. 'Hey yourself. How're you doing?'

His smile was wry. 'Not bad. I've had more fun Saturday nights though.'

I nodded gravely. 'Me too. How's Charlotte?'

He sighed. 'Not great, not sure whether she's done the right thing, questioning the friendship they had, worrying she'd led him on, worrying whether she was stupid to break things off.'

'It's so rotten. I honestly thought from seeing them together that they were both pretty smitten with each other.'

Adam nodded. 'I know. The thing is, I'm not sure Charlie's ever been that way with anyone. She's a very independent person. She's talking about going travelling for a bit to get her head clear.'

Charlotte's work as a trainer for computer software was on a contract basis and made for a lot of down time, which made travelling easy. She could easily take some time off for a month or two and pick things up afterwards. I just wasn't sure if that would make it easier or harder to move on.

Adam smiled. 'This gallivanting round the world at the end of a relationship might catch on.' Ah, his ex.

I looked at him closely, trying to figure out if there was any wistfulness there. I couldn't tell, so I decided the simplest thing to do was to ask.

'Any pangs on that score?'

He leaned down to kiss my nose and then put his arm round me.

'Absolutely not, Ms Morgan. In fact, the exact opposite.'

I smiled. 'Good answer.'

Charlotte didn't go away in the end. She didn't see Tom any more either, though. He was bereft at the break-up, and I felt much sympathy for him, not least because there were a lot of parallels with my break-up with James: the sense that it hadn't been a 'proper' relationship, whatever that was, but that it was more than a series of random hook-ups.

Honestly, the whole friends-with-benefits and fuck-buddy culture that seems to have become more *de rigueur* for our generation is a difficult world to navigate. For every relationship like the one I had with Tom (which ended organically, cleanly and with neither one of us feeling upset by the other), there were many others involving hurt feelings, misunderstandings and no bloody sense of where you stand with things. While I'd loved the experiences I'd had along the way and the chance to discover more about what I was into (and, of course, the inordinate amount of fun I'd had), I was most definitely happy that uncertainty was no longer an issue. I just hoped Tom would be able to move on and find his own happiness.

He was definitely not hanging around waiting to do so, though. After the first few weeks of moping he signed up for an online dating site and for Fetlife, a D/s-focused social network. While he still spoke about Charlotte sometimes, he began talking to women online, although he wasn't quite ready to take the next step. It sounded like he was having some flirty fun – I just wasn't sure if this was going to be the start of the kind of relationship he wanted. It can be hard to tell if people are what they seem online.

Adam, on the other hand, remained nothing if not transparent. Sometimes that was accidentally amusing – for example, he had a tendency to become so focused on work that he tuned out everything else and it was a case of waving food in front of him (or stripping naked, that worked too) to get him to break off from what he was doing. It was OK, though, I didn't take it personally. I felt secure enough in his love for me that the quirks of his personality just amused me.

Sometimes I found him genuinely surprising, though.

We'd gone out to the supermarket on a Saturday morning, at the end of one of those weeks that feels distressingly like it'll never end. Adam was distracted to the point of hilarity. He forgot his wallet, and we ended up forgetting the milk and having to go back for it. By the time he'd stood in the car park for over a minute, unable to find the car, I was laughing at him outright. I couldn't help it. He was smiling, too, so I figured I was safe.

On the drive home he took a wrong turn, taking us to a neighbourhood not too far from our flat – but far enough that I was looking quizzically at him as he pulled over.

'You OK?' I asked, half expecting his strange behaviour to be a sign that he was ill.

'Yeah, I'm fine,' he said, getting out of the car. I was confused, but I followed him.

We crossed the road. Adam walked up to the front gate of a small house, and said hello to a man waiting there. Apparently he was waiting for us. I smiled hello, but didn't really know what to say because I had no clue what was going on. We followed the man inside, while my brain whirred – was this a potential new client of Adam's? A friend? Why hadn't he mentioned anything?

When we got inside, everything slotted into place. The house was empty, there was no furniture anywhere, and as we stood in the hallway it became apparent we were here to have a look round.

The estate agent, who'd come to let us in, agreed to leave us to it, seemingly keen to make a phone call from the warmth of his car parked in the drive.

As the front door closed behind him, I turned to look at Adam, my glance questioning. Well, at least this explained why he was distracted.

'You didn't mention we were looking at houses today.'

He looked a bit sheepish. 'We aren't, not really. It's just, I saw this advertised in the local paper and looked it up online and it just seemed similar to what we'd been talking about.'

I grinned. We had spent a ridiculous amount of time discussing what our dream house would look like, mostly because it made the endless saving feel more worthwhile. We wanted a little house (well, we'd have been happy with a big house, but we had to be realistic), big windows and a kitchen big enough for a little table (me), room for a home office (both of us), all painted in neutral colours (him) but with lots of opportunities for shelves and bright sofas and the like (me). Preferably a little garden, mostly so that I could have a free-standing hammock (I know it's a ridiculous thing to fixate on, but honestly, a free-standing hammock to lie on while reading my Kindle is pretty much my summer-day dream) and Adam could have a barbecue.

I had no idea how much this would cost and no sense of whether this would or could become our home. But twenty minutes' dreaming about it wouldn't hurt anyone would it? I took his hand. 'Come on then, show me round.'

We went for a wander. A fairly short wander. Our budget did not stretch to a stately home. But as I walked into the living room and saw the big bay windows and the tiny conservatory out the back I felt a weird moment of recognition. I could imagine us living here. I could imagine Adam's herb pots on the kitchen window ledge, our DVD shelves in the nook by the living-room door, a little arm-chair in the conservatory where I could sit with my laptop to write – it'd be a suntrap in the summer and would echo with the sound of rain on the glass roof in winter, a cosy place to sit bundled up out of the poor weather. As we walked through the house I loved it more and more, could hear the voice of my dad – who had given us both lectures on the dangers of falling for a house and thus not getting the best deal because you were too emotional – warning me to stay calm and be objective.

By the time I saw the deep bath with a power shower over the top of it, I was gone. I snuck a look over at Adam. He seemed distracted still, but even he was impressed – the low pressure of our shower was a constant bugbear of his.

I had no idea what we did now. How this worked. I didn't even know if we could afford it. This was all grown-up stuff, new things I had no clue about, that we'd talked about but that now – maybe? – might be happening.

I walked over to the window in the master bedroom and looked out onto the garden shed. A shed. I laughed at myself, both for being excited at potentially having a shed and for not knowing what on earth I should put into one. I stood, watching a woman hanging out her washing a few doors down.

'What do you think?' Adam asked from across the room. 'They've priced it for a quick sale and they want buyers with no chain. We could put in a speculative offer at least.'

'I love it,' I said. 'I can imagine us living here.'

'There's room for us to have kids.'

I laughed. 'Kids plural? Hold on, I've not even set up a home office yet and we're talking about moving things round?'

He didn't respond to my mocking, his voice was suddenly serious. 'It'd be good to get married first, though, wouldn't it?'

I was still watching the woman. 'Before we have kids? I

suppose so, although if it happens the other way around that wouldn't be too much of a problem. We'd get there in the end.'

'I know, but it'd be better to be married, wouldn't it?'

I turned to look at him, and found him in a weird half-crouched position. He straightened up as I moved. For long moments neither of us said anything.

'Sophie, I'm trying to ask you to marry me.'

I was speechless. I literally couldn't speak. I didn't cry, I think I was too surprised. I know, we'd been talking about buying a home together, we already lived together, we wanted kids. I just hadn't expected it now, here.

We looked at each other. After a few more seconds he finally, and somewhat plaintively said, 'Soph? You're kind of leaving me hanging here.' I laughed.

'You haven't actually asked me to marry you yet.'

He looked confused. 'Yes I did.'

'No, you didn't. You said you were trying to, but you didn't.'

'You're such a bloody pedant.' I crossed my arms, although I think my massive grin probably gave away my feelings. He chuckled and bowed. 'Ms Sophie Morgan, will you marry me? Please?'

I couldn't stop myself getting a bit choked up then, although I drew the line at the weird flappy-hand thing women do in chick flicks. 'Of course I will. I'd love to.' A pause. Simpler? 'Yes.'

I flew across the room, launching myself at him. He half caught me, half hugged me, and we kissed for long enough that I was suddenly a bit worried the estate agent might come back. When we broke apart we were grinning at each other like lunatics, Adam's face visibly relieved. Well, I guess that explained his distraction.

Suddenly, Adam made a little noise of exclamation. 'Oh, I almost forgot.' He pulled a small box out of his pocket, and opened it to show me a ring.

'If you don't like it, or it doesn't fit, we can change it,' he said as he pulled it from the box and went to slip it on my finger. It was simple and not ostentatious, exactly the kind of the thing I would have chosen for myself. I hugged him tightly.

'It's perfect.'

He kissed me on the nose.

'You're perfect.'

I pulled a face. 'No I'm not.'

He grinned. 'OK, you're not perfect. You're argumentative for starters.'

I nodded. 'But you can be incredibly smug at times.'

He feigned thought. 'OK, I'll let you have that. But you're stubborn.'

I was outraged. 'So are you!'

He kissed me again. 'That's not the point. The point is, you're perfect for me.'

I looked up at him and felt a surge of love for my good-hearted, loving, clever, funny, kind, filthy and twisted Adam. 'You're perfect for me too.'

And he really was.

Epilogue

Everyone has their favourite places to be. The beach, Disney World, the terrace of their favourite team's ground, maybe just surrounded by family and friends at home. I love all those places (albeit I'm the very definition of a fair-weather sports fan), but one of my favourite places to be is in bed with Adam.

I know. You've just read 300-plus pages about how much I enjoy that, so it's not a shocker to you.

But when we climb into bed and curl up together, I feel safe, happy, loved, at home, in a way that I never did before. It's not the bed, or the duvet or even the room itself. It's the man behind me, literally and figuratively, whose dominance reflects back my submission, even while we go through our daily life as partners. Equals.

That's not to say work and other responsibilities, the detritus of real life, don't get in the way sometimes. Not all the sex we have is full-on D/s sex. That's not a bad thing – variety is the spice of live after all, and after a while even the loveliest things can get a bit samey. There's little risk of that for us, though, not least because we've got plenty of toys and outfits we've accrued along the way to make it fun when we have the time and inclination to let loose.

But sometimes there are no outfits. No floggers. No expanding butt plugs. There's just us. And those are the most intimate times of all.

He lies behind me, pressed close into my back, one of his arms under my neck and the other wrapped around my body in a kind of backwards cuddle, most of my body (or all the important bits for our purposes) within his reach. His head is close to mine, so when he whispers in my ear, the feeling of his breath on my neck makes me shiver.

Often as we lie like this he'll tell me dirty stories. We'll talk about things we've done together, things we might like to try, things we wouldn't want to do in real life but which are hot to talk about, lying in bed in the dark. Sometimes when we lie here, in our little cocoon, making each other squirm with lust at the stories we're weaving together, Adam's hand will snake between my legs and play with me until I am desperate to come, my legs shaking with the effort of holding off my orgasm.

Not tonight, though. Not yet anyway. The thing is, he is still much more patient than me. He begins a dirty story, a variation on one we've talked about before – a fantasy that logistically is pretty unlikely to come to fruition. As he speaks, he strokes my arm with his fingertips, punctuating his sentences with kisses and nibbling on my ear, neck and shoulder. All of which, of course, drives me crazy and makes me wet.

Some days he would be fine with my hand sliding between my own legs. Some days he would actively encourage it and quite enjoy watching. Not tonight, though, tonight he definitely disapproves of my attempt to relieve my building sexual tension. As soon as he realises where my hand is going, he grabs my wrist.

'Not yet.'

I make a grumbling noise as he pulls my arm away and continues with what he had been doing.

'And you can cut out that attitude as well.' His voice is amused, mostly, but has the edge of steel to it that, even now, gives me butterflies.

'I don't have an attitude.' I know, I'm not helping myself by answering back. But some days he is so bloody smug. I know it's not breaking news, but even so.

He stops his touching and kissing and lifts his head up away from me for a moment.

'I'm being perfectly nice to you right now, all you need to do is show some patience and lie back and appreciate it a little bit.'

I consider my position. Is it worth arguing and risking the consequences? Probably not. But I'm not happy. As ever, some days the submissive mindset is one that comes down as quickly as a fog on a wintry day, while at other points I have the urge to rebel, even though I know that not only is this a game that I can't win, it's a game that I actively don't want to win.

His voice has taken on the slight sing-song timbre that makes me want to kneel at his feet and kick him in the shins in about equal measure – although obviously doing both at the same time is somewhat impractical.

'You should know by now, if you'd asked permission to touch yourself it would have been much more effective.'

I stay quiet but, fortunately for me, the bedside light has already been turned off so he can't see my face. If he did I'd probably be told off for glaring at him.

He goes back to teasing me. No spanking or further

humiliation, yet, but I know he's making it last longer than he otherwise would have done to teach me a lesson.

Finally his hand is on my inner thigh. By now I'm so turned on I am starting to shiver. I feel him laugh behind me, which doesn't help my grumpy face. When he finally runs his finger along my wetness I can't suppress my low moan of pleasure.

'You see, here's the problem. Even now, after all this time, there are some days where your brain wants to fight me and makes you angry with me. You're confused here –' he tapped my head with his other hand, even while his fingers pushed deeper between my legs, causing me to swallow a sigh of pleasure. He chuckled. 'You're not confused here. This is the truth. This shows how much you love this. All of it. This is why you need to think with your cunt and not with your brain – you'll be much happier.'

I wonder if now is the point to make a smart comment about blokes thinking with their cocks. I'm guessing not.

As he finishes his lecture he pushes a finger inside me. I gasp and blush. I am wet, oh so wet, but I am also furious, although I honestly can't tell you if it's at him or myself.

'So fucking smug.' The words slip out. I snap my mouth shut, half hoping that I can swallow back my outburst.

No such luck.

'What did you say?' His response is quick and sharp.

'Nothing.'

'Don't fib. You said something about smug.'

I call him smug all the time. He certainly doesn't mind me mocking him, but these things are always about context. In this situation, at this moment, he isn't going to let me get away with anything.

Eventually, somewhat sheepishly, I repeat myself. In an instant his fingers are gone, his palm resting just above my wetness. He is unmoving. No kissing, no stroking, no more whispering. His arm is still under my neck, but he has released my breast, which he had been caressing.

Silence.

I am nervous. Aroused. Curious. Will he hurt me in some way? But he doesn't. He just lies there, letting the silence grow. I don't know if it's one minute or ten, but it seems to drag on and on.

Finally he speaks. 'It's quite the battle of wills we have going on here, isn't it?'

'I don't know what you mean,' I reply. I do.

'I've been nothing but nice to you but, because I'm not going at the speed that you want, you want things all your own way.'

I bite back a retort about things fundamentally being all his way, mostly because I know that's actually not true, that we both enjoy this, that there is still equality of pleasure in this inequality, that for some reason I have brattier urges than usual today.

As the silence lengthens I worry I've disappointed him. I hate that. I feel my resolve melt away. It takes a little longer before I can respond, but I finally find my voice.

'I'm sorry, I'll be good.'

His fingers are back as quickly as they had gone. Stroking me, spreading my lips apart and dipping inside me.

'You know that you're wetter now than when I stopped?'

It takes all the effort I can muster not to call him smug

again. I settle for mentally calling him an arse, and am once again thankful that he can't see my face.

He doesn't stop talking, though. His voice becomes a constant whisper in my ear.

'This is what I'm talking about. Stop thinking with your head, think a little more with this.' His fingers move inside me. 'It always knows what you want to do, what you enjoy, even when your stubborn brain hasn't caught up yet. That's why this cunt belongs to me.'

I moan in spite of myself.

'That's it, let go, just be a good girl for me. You clearly want to, don't you?'

My blood begins to sing, my body reacts to his. I feel my submission wash over me and as I offer it to him, I become pliant beneath him.

It's a game we've played so often before, that we'll undoubtedly play over and over again, hopefully for the rest of our lives. It is intense, fun, arousing, amazing.

His fingers move between my legs, punctuating his whispered lecture about how much I enjoy this, how we both know that I love this, live for it at times, especially when he's got his hand between my legs.

It makes me blush, but we both know that it's the truth. My hips are arching as I press my swollen clit into his hand – it's something of a giveaway.

As I get close to coming he slows his movements. I bite back a moan, knowing that it will get me into trouble, instead leaving myself in his hands, on his timescale. He nods in approval behind me.

'Good girl. Trust me to look after you. Be patient.'

I feel a flush of warmth at the praise, and a flash of

affection for him. He does look after me, sexually and otherwise. Suddenly I feel the proper rush of the apology I had given grudgingly before.

'I'm sorry. I shouldn't have said you were smug.'

He chuckles behind me. 'Oh, sweetheart, I am smug.'

I restrain the urge to nod, not sure if I'm safe doing that yet and not willing to risk it.

'But the thing is, even though I am smug, sometimes I like having a reason to punish you, and your outburst gives me that reason.'

My heart begins to beat even faster. It's not fear, though, it's anticipation. I am smiling as I speak. 'As long as you're not ever hoping I'm going to be the kind of submissive who stops mocking you and obeys your every whim.'

He shifts me onto my front for a moment, running his hand along the curve of my arse. I am smiling in the darkness as he begins to spank the place where my arse meets the top of my thighs, the sweet spot that makes me squirm.

'I'm very happy with the mocking. And let's face it, we both know I don't need a reason to punish you, that's not how this works.' He is warming my cheek, his spanking gentle as he allows me to get used to the feeling of his hand connecting with my arse. Even after all this time it is one of the most intimate things we do, and the feeling of his palm connecting, the intimacy of his touch, makes me sigh. It's a happy sound.

The warmth on my cheek at the sting of his slaps is beginning to build as I adjust to the pain. I nod my agreement, taking deep breaths through my nose, trying to conquer the pain, ride the endorphin rush. He hits me harder, and I squirm, urging my arse up to meet his hand. Eager.

By the time he moves me back against him, I can feel his erection pressing into me and he can feel the heat of my punished cheek against his thigh. He sighs in satisfaction and nips my shoulder with his teeth, before he moves his hand between my legs and begins spanking there. I push my hips upwards, meeting him eagerly, so eagerly he chuckles.

I love this. We both do. I'm past the point of feeling like I need to apologise for it. We're not hurting anyone else, we're doing it safely. It's all consensual. He knows me well, sometimes it feels he knows me better than I know myself – although, yes, I'm better at using my safe word nowadays.

This makes my nipples hard, it makes me wet. The challenge, the fight, being overpowered, being tied up, being hurt. Yielding to him, pleasing him, loving him. It all meshes together in my brain – the pain with the pleasure, the adrenaline with the endorphins. Most times the fight isn't literal, but we are vying for power and I love the intimacy of it, the control he has. Sometimes I give him that control willingly, sometimes he takes it, albeit still with my permission. Either way I enjoy it, enjoy him, enjoy being on the back foot, not knowing what is going to happen next.

Reacting. Enduring. Enjoying.

I love him. I love it.